P9-ASE-130

GREAT WRITERS STUDENT LIBRARY

# RESTORATION
# AND
# 18th-CENTURY
# DRAMA

# GREAT WRITERS STUDENT LIBRARY

Editor: James Vinson
Associate Editor: D. L. Kirkpatrick

GREAT WRITERS OF THE ENGLISH LANGUAGE

# RESTORATION

# AND

# 18th-CENTURY

# DRAMA

INTRODUCTION BY

ARTHUR H. SCOUTEN

ST. MARTIN'S PRESS
NEW YORK

© The Macmillan Press Ltd., 1980

All rights reserved. For more information,
write:
St. Martin's Press, Inc.
175 Fifth Avenue,
New York, NY 10010

Printed in Hong Kong

First published in the United States of
America in 1980

Scouten: *Restoration and 18th Century Drama*

ISBN 0-312-34704-9

**Library of Congress Number:**
79-5249

# CONTENTS

# EDITOR'S NOTE

The entry for each writer consists of a biography, a complete list of his published books, a selected list of published bibliographies and critical studies on the writer, and a signed critical essay on his work.

In the biographies, details of education, military service, and marriage(s) are generally given before the usual chronological summary of the life of the writer; awards and honours are given last.

The Publications section is meant to include all book publications, though as a rule broadsheets, single sermons and lectures, minor pamphlets, exhibition catalogues, etc. are omitted. Under the heading Collections, we have listed the most recent collections of the complete works and those of individual genres (verse, plays, novels, stories, and letters); only those collections which have some editorial authority and were issued after the writer's death are listed; on-going editions are indicated by a dash after the date of publication; often a general selection from the writer's works or a selection from the works in the individual genres listed above is included.

Titles are given in modern spelling, though the essayists were allowed to use original spelling for titles and quotations; often the titles are "short." The date given is that of the first book publication, which often followed the first periodical or anthology publication by some time; we have listed the actual year of publication, often different from that given on the title-page. No attempt has been made to indicate which works were published anonymously or pseudonymously, or which works of fiction were published in more than one volume. We have listed plays which were produced but not published, but only since 1700; librettos and musical plays are listed along with the other plays; no attempt has been made to list lost or unverified plays. Reprints of books (including facsimile editions) and revivals of plays are not listed unless a revision or change of title is involved. The most recent edited version of individual works is included if it supersedes the collected edition cited.

In the essays, short references to critical remarks refer to items cited in the Publications section or in the Reading List. Introductions, memoirs, editorial matter, etc. in works cited in the Publications section are not repeated in the Reading List.

# INTRODUCTION

From 1660 to 1800 there appeared a body of dramatic literature, frequently scorned in the 19th and early 20th centuries, that has found increasing appreciation in modern times. It was once the dull duty of the literary historian (often a specialist in Elizabethan drama) to comment on the immorality and licentiousness of the Restoration comedies as he proceeded to chronicle the decay and downfall of English drama, but a look at recent bibliographies or publishers' advertisements will show the remarkable increase of editions of these plays and the general respect being accorded by modern critics. The dramatic works by the authors during this one hundred and forty year period are so diverse in nature that they prove recalcitrant to easy categorization. To avoid broad generalisations which would scarcely be valid for so many writers over such a long period of time, I will break my account into three sections: the reign of Charles II, 1660–1685; 1685 until the Stage Licensing Act of 1737; and 1737 until 1800, or thereabouts.

As Robert Hume points out in his important study, *The Development of English Drama in the Late Seventeenth Century,* literary historians have not yet been able to establish a terminal date for Restoration drama. Most of them set the period from 1660 to 1700, using the premiere of *The Way of the World* as the culmination of the type of play called the comedy of manners. Others want to include Farquhar and hence extend the date to 1707, the year of *The Beaux Stratagem,* and some push the terminus three more years, to include the retirement of Thomas Betterton, the great actor-manager who had performed in many of the major successes of the age. Finally, John Loftis, the editor of the Nebraska Regents series of reprints, stretched the period to 1737. This extension led of course to ludicrous difficulties. In one case, a critic, who shall be nameless here, called Susannah Centlivre's *The Busy Body* (1709) a lively Restoration comedy, but classified Nicholas Rowe's farce *The Biter* (1704) as "a tedious eighteenth century play." Hence I will be a strict constructionist and apply the term "Restoration" to those plays, lively or tedious, which were acted after the restoration of good King Charles to the English throne.

The year 1737 provides a valid dividing point for the second section, as the Stage Licensing Act ended the theatrical career of Henry Fielding and the experimental dramatists whose innovative plays he had been staging. Furthermore, a number of years passed after 1737 before new, full-length plays were produced; thus there is a real, though brief, break in continuity.

## 1. The Drama from 1660 to 1685

The major rupture of continuity, of course, was the eighteen-year cessation of acting during the interregnum. The result of this hiatus was that most of the new Restoration plays differed so considerably from those of the Elizabethan period that historians have not been able to agree on the relative importance of the different causes of the change. Some account, then, should be given of the influence of contemporary French drama, the burden of Italian and French Neoclassic theories, trends in Caroline drama, the vogue of the Spanish Romance, and the historical and social background of the literary scene in the 1660's.

Years ago, when Restoration comedy was in disrepute, its emergence was attributed to the influence of French drama, thereby removing a stain from the purity of English literature. From the record of new plays in London during the first decade of the restoration of the monarchy, we can see that this ascription is fallacious, in so far as comedy is concerned. Much has been made of English borrowings from Molière, but the essential form of the new satiric wit-comedy characteristic of Restoration drama had already been established by the time of *The Misanthrope* and *Tartuffe* in 1666 and 1667.

Royalist exiles waiting in Paris for Oliver Cromwell to die did have the opportunity to see tragedies by Corneille and admire the emphasis placed on *gloire* and on loyalty to the monarch. They also became accustomed to the musical and psychological effects of the rhymed alexandrine couplet. Furthermore, all persons interested in literature, whether expatriates or quietly living in England, were becoming conversant with the propositions concerning dramatic literature propounded by French Neoclassic critics. The goal of perfecting tragedy by moving it in the direction of the epic (the queen of literary forms) was most attractive, and even before 1660 we find English writers such as Hobbes and Davenant speculating on this topic. Besides, Englishmen visiting Paris or the northern Italian cities were impressed by the spectacle incorporated into the staging of tragedies and operas. Hence we can see that a potential audience was already being prepared for the heroic play when English dramatists came to compose them. English devotees of the theatre evinced great interest in the introduction of rhymed verse for the language of tragedy. The campaign being carried out in Paris to refine, correct, polish, and preserve the French language could not fail to impress English observers, who soon realised that this mode provided a route whereby they could surpass the literary giants of the Elizabethan age, "the race before the flood." All these points are discussed at length by John Dryden in his *Essay of Dramatic Poesy*, the best introduction to Restoration Drama that has ever been written.

The attractiveness of the heroic play was further enhanced by the active support of Charles II himself. He too had seen the French serious dramas in Paris, certainly not overlooking their support of the values of a hierarchical society, and he suggested to Roger Boyle, Earl of Orrery, the composition of such a play. Later, when productions of the heroic drama were under way, he and his brother, the Duke of York, not only brought the court to attend performances but also lent royal robes to the actors for costumes. When we add to these influential forces at work the fact that "love-and-honour" plays had previously been acted for Queen Henrietta Marie and her court in the time of Charles I and thus had already become part of the native tradition in serious drama, we should be prepared for an early advent of the heroic play on the London stage.

The first one, *The General*, was composed in 1661 by Lord Orrery, and first performed in Dublin in 1662. However, the first heroic play witnessed by a London audience was *The Indian Queen*, a collaboration of Sir Robert Howard and John Dryden, in January 1664. It was followed immediately by Orrery's *The History of Henry the Fifth* in August of that year, and others by Dryden, Orrery, Elkanah Settle, John Caryl, and Samuel Pordage appeared in the next few years. The wild rant and extravagant action in these plays make them objectionable, worse yet, even ludicrous to the modern reader. Accordingly, to understand the admiration which the original audiences had for these plays, we must remember Erich Auerbach's explanation in *Mimesis* of the fascination which the courtiers had for works which presented the crisis of leaders, torn by contrary demands from their private life and their duties as rulers.

The other major influence on the new dramatists came from Spain. The borrowed elements are relatively novel and can be easily traced as they appear. One feature was a highly complicated plot, giving rise, in English hands, to a sub-genre which Allardyce Nicoll termed "intrigue plays." Of the borrowed character types, the Spanish fathers turn out to be unusually choleric and bombastic, the young male leads are haughty though idealistic, but it is the high-spirited heroines who set the tone of the work. These young ladies are both virtuous and loquacious. They object wittily and vociferously to marriages which their fathers have arranged, but they are women of high moral fibre and while they talk audaciously, they never say anything indecent. Their high moral standards do not lead them to a submissive attitude in the presence of their suitors; instead, the young ladies engage in a free, open, and even equal basis, and are ready to out-talk any man who starts an argument. The initial English use of this material appeared in the first major box-office success of the Restoration period, *The Adventures of Five Hours* (1663), by Sir Samuel Tuke. Pepys and other commentators quickly noticed both the liveliness of the play and the complete lack of anything bawdy. The playwrights soon employed the Spanish romance to their advantage. In *The Carnival,* Thomas Porter presents the young male lead and the heroine as the two main characters, rather than designating the man as the protagonist, and achieves what John Harrington Smith was later to call "the gay couple." This achievement of an almost complete equality of the sexes engaged in a duel of wits came to be the distinguishing sign of Restoration comedy. Dryden saw that all he needed to add was some racy language to the women's parts, and he would have perfect material for the theatre – especially when the actress was Nell Gwyn. The best example of the dramatic possibilities is found in the famous encounter between Dorimant and Harriet in Etherege's *The Man of Mode* (1676).

This presentation of foreign elements does not mean that there was no connection between the new drama and the old. The break with Elizabethan tragedy was complete, but various aspects of the older comedy continued on in the Restoration plays. Fletcher's comedies were at the peak of their reputation in the 1660's; they were offered frequently in the theatre and were imitated by young playwrights. In contrast to the exphasis on action and complicated plot-turns in the Spanish plays, Fletcher's comedies put the major emphasis on dialogue. The last Caroline plays before the outbreak of war blossomed again in the Restoration, especially festive comedies like Brome's *The Jovial Crew,* whose cheerful and optimistic tone is perpetuated in the newly-discovered *The Country Gentleman,* by Sir Robert Howard and George Villiers, 2nd Duke of Buckingham. But the most influential of all the Elizabethan writers was Ben Jonson. We mistake the true nature of his influence if we seek only for some Restoration comedies containing "humors" characters. Jonson's use of humors characters was only a device; the medical metaphor was outmoded in the late seventeenth century anyhow; and the members of the *dramatis personae* labelled with a "humor" in some Restoration plays are actually "social" types (fop, rake, cast-off mistress) rather than humor characters. Nor is the adulation lavished on the name of Ben Jonson a reliable sign. Almost everyone, it appears, praised him, but they went to see Shakespeare's plays in the theatres. The recorded number of performances of Jonson's comedies in the years 1660–1700 is very low, and not at all in line with the number of allusions to him in essays, prologues, poems, and the like.

The true relation between Ben Jonson's comedies and most Restoration comedies is that both share the same pessimistic view of the nature of man and his hostility toward his fellow man; both demonstrate an unceasing animosity between the different social classes; and both sets of comedies modulate toward being open-ended. To illustrate the difference from Elizabethan or eighteenth-century comedy, we can invoke Shakespeare. At the beginning of his comedy *The Tempest,* practically everybody is hostile to some other person or group; plots and counter-plots abound. But by the end of the play, everyone but Caliban realises that there is a universal harmony; everyone becomes reconciled and Prospero can break his staff. Again, what could exceed the hostility shown in *The Merchant of Venice?* Yet all is resolved in universal harmony at Belmont. But when we turn to Ben Jonson's *The Alchemist,* the play just stops. The cleverest rascal gets off, scotfree, and there is little doubt he will ply his trade again. So too in Sir Robert Howard's charming comedy *The Committee* (1662). Here, the demure heroine Ruth blackmails the greedy, social climbing Puritan Mrs. Day into a stalemate, without any resolution. The Puritans (in the play) still control England; they hate the Royalists and seek to humiliate them as well as take their estates; the frustrated Cavaliers return the hatred. *The Country-Wife* (1675) ends when Margery Pinchwife is corrupted; the dance stops with the music, and will resume when the musicians start playing again, but the hostility between Horner and Pinchwife has not the least abated. *The Man of Mode* stops when Dorimant agrees to visit Harriet's country home, but the play presents no resolution. This open-ended nature of the structure of much Restoration comedy certainly proclaims the debt to the master satirist Ben Jonson.

As can be seen from the presentation of the Puritans in Howard's *The Committee,* the historical and social background had much to do in shaping the nature of early Restoration drama. To the young people of the 1660's, the recent Civil War was a monstrous stroke of folly. The events in it and the conduct of the leaders showed that older people were incapable of running the country properly, and that no one should pay the least attention to the elderly anyhow. The recently-found comedy *The Country Gentleman* does treat an older man in a favorable light, but otherwise the situation in Restoration comedies of the 1660's was the same as in Paris in May 1968 – no one over thirty was fit to be trusted.

The "noble experiment" of Puritan rule was regarded with cynicism. After they had won the civil war, the Puritan leaders, proud of their high ethics, determined not to confiscate captured property as conquerors throughout history had done; instead, they set up sequestration courts and committees. However, if a Royalist nobleman returned to claim his property, he might find himself executed or jailed. Most of the Cavaliers lacked cash to pay their taxes, and saw their estates pass into the greedy hands of the sequestration committees, so that either way the loyal supporters of the Stuarts lost their lands. Nor was the Restoration settlement acceptable all around. To regain one's property, a man needed money and lawyers for the long rounds in the law courts. Many Londoners bitterly resented the return of Charles II, and there were several abortive revolts. This situation made the Stuart supporters nervous, ill-tempered, and reckless, so that hedonism became the vogue.

It is not surprising then to see the new young playwrights hit back at the Puritans. No later than Charles's return, and possibly slightly before, John Tatham brought out his vindictive satire, *The Rump,* presenting the frenzied scrambles first for power and then for safety on the part of the deceased Cromwell's lieutenants. This piece was followed in 1661 by the poet Cowley's satire on the Puritans, *Cutter of Coleman Street.* In 1662 came Howard's *The Committee,* the best of the group, followed in the next year by John Wilson's *The Cheats* and John Lacy's *The Old Troop.* These were the first new plays of the Restoration, not the celebrated wit comedies or sex comedies.

Another factor affecting the playwrights and the development of the drama was the audience. In 1600, when London was a city of from 150,000 to possibly 200,000 people, the drama was at the height of its popularity, and despite the opposition to the theatre by the Puritans, the city was able to support six or seven established theatrical troupes. In 1660, the King issued two licenses (to Davenant and Killigrew) to create a monopoly, and itinerant troupes were crushed or absorbed. Thus until nearly the end of Charles's reign, the city of London, now with a population of about 400,000, was only barely maintaining two theatrical companies. In spite of royal patronage, the two companies did not prosper uniformly, and by 1682 the King's Company had lost so much money that it was ended, with the players being absorbed by the Duke's company. Thus in the last three years of Charles's reign, and on into 1695, only one company was staging plays.

Not only had the drama lost its popular base, as the chief form of entertainment for Londoners, but the bulk of the remaining theatregoers constituted a coterie audience. It is true that in recent years closer study of the evidence has shown that some business men, clerks, and servants occasionally attended the theatre, but the great majority of the regular audience were members of the court, or lesser figures in government administration, or other members of the upper middle class, or the law students. The result was that the dramatists were no longer writing for a large, heterogeneous audience, and the new plays were designed for this smaller coterie audience. Accordingly, many of the plays were highly topical and included specific, personal satire.

This brief survey of the main influences on the new playwrights has already dealt with several of the emerging types of drama: the heroic play, intrigue comedy, the beginnings of wit comedy, and the political plays. What remains now is to focus on the main lines of development in comedy and tragedy. Though the new comedies each season exhibited considerable variety, a type was developing which has been called wit comedy or the comedy of manners. Dryden took the lead, as he had with the heroic drama, and presented a gay couple in *The Wild Gallant* (1663) and an even more vivacious pair in *Secret Love* (1667). James Sutherland points out that the playwright James Howard contributed two plays, *The English Monsieur* and *All Mistaken,* in the pattern which evolved into the comedy of manners. The first two plays of George Etherege are more instructive in showing us what happened. Into the first, *The Comical Revenge* (1664), Etherege crammed four plots, with the *dramatis personae* for each drawn from a different class of London society. The first complication concerns noblemen who had participated in the Civil War, and is in the context of the love-and-honour heroic drama. The main plot presents a rake and a widow, both from the upper middle class. The third group comprises of gamblers, sharpers, and their victim, and the last episode deals with servants. A just treatment of these several lines would require a novel, possibly in more than one volume. Whether Etherege saw this problem or not, he turned his focus of interest to one group in his next play – *She Wou'd If She Cou'd* (1668) – the members of middle-class London society. The protagonist is a rake who is looking out for sexual experiences while pursuing his main goal – marriage to a rich heiress. Looking backwards through the drama, we can see that Etherege fixed the group to be dealt with in this art form, and the group he presented is in the same category as those ever since, in the comedy of manners, down through Oscar Wilde and Somerset Maugham. Etherege was an objective observer, and William Wycherley, now looked on as the best comic dramatist among this early group, introduced more satiric drive in his plays. Because of the virulent satire in *The Country-Wife* (1675) and *The Plain-Dealer* (1676), this type of Restoration play is often called satiric comedy. The first wave of the comedy of manners reached its peak in 1676, with the production in that year of *The Plain-Dealer,* Etherege's polished masterpiece, *The Man of Mode,* and Shadwell's satire on the dabblers in science, *The Virtuoso.* No one knew it at the time but the artistic achievement of these plays marked the close of the first wave of the comedy of manners. Wycherley and Etherege had written their last play, and the next group of comic dramatists took comedy in a different direction. Tom D'Urfey and Aphra Behn began a series of racy plays which we may call sex-comedy, marked by the bawdy language so offensive to our Victorian ancestors. Dryden, who should have known better, composed a play of this type, *Mr. Limberham* (1678), which proved quite a shocker, in spite of Dryden's protest that he was writing satire. At any rate, the comedies of the next few years certainly degenerated in dramatic quality, regardless of whether the reader is amused or offended by the indecency of language and situation. Comedy, which had gotten off to such a promising start in the 1660's, was in a decline by the end of Charles's reign.

Meanwhile, the progress of tragedy was following a different route. From the beginning, the artificiality of the heroic drama had led to objections and eventually to a diminution of audience interest. Also, other poets could not equal the nervous rhymed couplets of Dryden's plays. Dryden himself wearied of the heroic play and turned away from it. A period of experimentation went on, with mediocre authors like Settle reviving the old revenge play. Then two able playwrights appeared in the persons of Thomas Otway and Nathaniel Lee. Both turned to the high road of English tragedy – tragedy of character. Neither was entirely successful, but Otway achieved the best tragedy of the entire period under consideration in this volume, *Venice Preserved* (1682), and Lee's *The Rival Queens* (1677) held the stage for over a century and a half. Dryden himself showed renewed vitality in the tragic form with *All for Love* (1677) and *Don Sebastian* (though the latter play was held back and not acted until 1689). An initial conclusion then would indicate that after the delay occasioned by the false start with the heroic play, English tragedy was on the way to new heights. Unfortunately, Otway died in 1684, poor Nathaniel Lee lost his senses and was committed to Bedlam in 1684, and the renewal of tragic form proved to be temporary and illusory. Worse yet, a minor playwright, John Banks, was to alter the nature of contemporary tragedy by abandoning the tragic hero. The process of enervating the male lead had been begun by Dryden in his depiction of Antony's degeneration in *All for Love,* and Castalio in Otway's *The Orphan* (1680) and Jaffeir in *Venice Preserved* are both weaklings. But John Banks completely subordinated the hero in *The Unhappy Favourite,* in 1681, and arranged for the women to take over. In the next year, he wrote *Anna Bullen,* where a weak, vacillating woman is the main character. Contemporary critics sneered and termed the plays "she-tragedies," but the damage was done. With the beautiful and tender Anne Bracegirdle available for the role, dramatists now composed tragedies featuring a tender woman in distress. The consequence was that the quality of tragedy plummeted rapidly.

With the prevailing cynicism of the age, it is not surprising to find the emergence of burlesque and farce. The sceptics had rejected the heroic play from the beginning, and the Duke of Buckingham, aided by several friends, put all the objections to bad drama together to create *The Rehearsal* (1671). More lively burlesque came from the pen of Thomas Duffett, as he pounced on Settle in *The Empress of Morocco* (1673) and on the attempts to create dramatic opera in his *The Mock-Tempest* (1674) and *Psyche Debauched* (1675).

Farcical episodes were prevalent in Elizabethan drama, but in the Restoration period authors began systematically to compose full-length five-act farces. The popularity of the *commedia dell'arte* led John Lacy, Nahum Tate, and Edward Ravenscroft, among others, to plunder these improvised comedies of the strolling Italian companies for use on the London stage. The most popular of all of the Restoration farces was Ravenscroft's *Mamamouchi* (1672), adapted and completely Englished from Molière. The most notorious full-length farce was Ravenscroft's *The London Cuckolds* (1681), where the hostility of the dramatists towards the London business men is made explicit. Much of the contents are pure slapstick comedy, and the play eschews the double-entendre and smutty talk of such comedies as *Mr. Limberham*. Ravenscroft drew upon both European folklore and scenes from Elizabethan comedy as sources for his amusing *lazzi* in this play. There was a good deal of contemporary commentary about the new mode of full-length farce, and Dryden and Shadwell got into a controversy over farce. Nahum Tate even wrote a serious justification of farce, as a preface to his successful assay, *A Duke and No Duke* (1684). The Lord Chamberlain's records show Charles II in frequent attendance at farces, and we can draw upon the irony implicit in this datum of fact to close this introduction to the development of drama in the time of this monarch.

## 2. The Drama from 1685 to 1737

English dramatists would never again enjoy as strong a royal patron as the Merry Monarch had been. It is true that his successor, James II, sponsored the drama, but he was out of office in three years, and William and Mary were not devotees of the theatre. Queen Anne would protect the players because of traditional Stuart support of the stage, but she took little interest in it. The Brunswick Georges preferred opera. For whom then would the dramatists write? It was the conjecture of John Harrington Smith that they tried to please "the Ladies," and that this change led to the introduction of sentimental elements (though Smith preferred the term "exemplary comedy" as a more accurate label for such plays). Unfortunately, we cannot be sure about the constituency of this new audience because of the numerous signs that the composition of the audience was changing. The first of these signals was lack of success for new plays for which great expectations had been entertained: Southerne's important comedy, *The Wives Excuse* (1691), failed on the night of its premiere. This mishap was followed by what might be called a general audience revolt at the turn of the century. Beginning in the autumn of 1697, almost all the new plays at both theatres were failures. Some fifteen new plays failed in this season of 1697–98, a disaster previously unheard of in theatre history. This rejection of new plays lasted for about six seasons, reaching a total of about seventy failures. What complicates the matter still more is the great variety in the kinds of dramas which were not being accepted. Congreve's artistic masterpiece, *The Way of the World,* achieved only a few performances, probably a total of six, when people in the theatre world expected a smash hit. In the same month, March 1700, William Burnaby's cynical and satiric comedy of manners, *The Reformed Wife,* also failed and had to be withdrawn. The contemporary play which we might consider at the furthest extreme of difference from these two comedies was Sir Richard Steele's whining, sentimental opus *The Lying Lover* (1703); yet it too was rejected and had to be dropped. A further sign of uncertainty in the audience was the failure of plays which later enjoyed great success. In 1703, Rowe's new tragedy, *The Fair Penitent,* failed, though it was in the new style of having a distressed heroine as the chief character in the play. It was revived in 1715, and went on to become one of the six or eight most popular tragedies of the century. The same pattern held for Colley Cibber's comedy *She Would and She Would*

*Not.* This play just barely reached a sixth night in November 1702, with such a small audience on the last night that the play was withdrawn. It was attempted again in 1707, when it again failed. Revived in 1714, it went on to become one of the most frequently acted plays on record, both in longevity and in total performances. Cibber's *Richard III* also failed in 1699 when it was first presented, and all students of the drama are generally aware of the tremendous and prolonged success that this adaptation from Shakespeare later enjoyed.

Proof that the composition of the audience was changing and that this pattern of theatrical failures did not arise from the antipathy of theatre-goers against a particular dramatist or type of play can be found in the surprising phenomenon of changing hours for the commencement of theatrical performances. For the convenience of the leisure class, plays throughout the Restoration had begun at four o'clock in the afternoon. The theatre is a relatively conservative institution, and starting times, once established, are rarely changed. However, from 1700 to 1705, the two playhouses began to push the opening time back, albeit irregularly, to four-thirty, then five, and sometimes to as late as six-thirty. From apologies in the newspapers and new advertisements announcing a four-thirty or five o'clock opening, we can infer that veteran theatre-goers had been protesting against the new hours, but subsequent playbills then announce the later hour of five-thirty or six. Such reversals certainly indicate an unstable situation and a changing audience.

I have presented this dreary and melancholy account (which can be studied fully in *The London Stage*) not to give a history of the period but to show the effect upon the dramatists. Let us see what happened. Thomas Southerne stopped writing comedies and wrote tragedies instead. Farquhar joined the army and was absent from the stage for three or four years. Vanbrugh turned his attention to architecture and stopped writing plays. But the most important withdrawal was that of William Congreve. It was Congreve who had revived the drama and whose sparkling comedies, *The Old Batchelor* (1693) and *Love for Love* (1695), had drawn large crowds to the theatre and had gotten the new company at Lincoln's Inn Fields off to a flying start. When *The Way of the World* did not answer expectations, Congreve stopped his playwriting. It would be difficult to exaggerate the severe consequences on English comedy caused by these withdrawals. When Wycherley and Etherege stopped composing plays, other, less able writers kept supplying the theatres with new plays, even if the quality was lowered. The withdrawal of a major dramatist – Congreve – and two excellent practitioners, Southerne and Vanbrugh, left only Farquhar. After his early death in 1707, there were not enough remaining playwrights of real ability, and comedy withered and declined.

After this general account of conditions in the theatre world at the beginning of the eighteenth century, it is time to trace the main directions of tragedy and comedy. The serious drama was now moving definitely in the direction of pathetic tragedy, with Southerne's *The Fatal Marriage* (1694) and Nicholas Rowe's *Jane Shore* (1714) becoming the most successful examples of the numerous attempts in this mode. Close study of the new tragedies, season by season, reveals authorial anxiety over the language of tragedy. Some writers even tried to revive the high-flown diction and rhymed couplets of the heroic play. D'Urfey went so far as to write his ten-act, two part *The Famous History of the Rise and Fall of Massaniello* (1699) in prose, a major break with convention. The full impact of the influence of neoclassic dramatic theory and of Racine came in the 1690's and the early eighteenth century. The results were meagre, as no plays of genuine dramatic tension appeared. The one real stage success was Addison's *Cato,* but its favorable reception came from an ideological basis, not an aesthetic one. The later neoclassic plays became increasingly derivative, with the last prominent example, Aaron Hill's *Zara* (1735), being adapted from Voltaire.

However, just as tragedy seemed at its nadir, a brief revival came in an attempt to restore domestic tragedy. Yet even the six or seven new plays in this style were clumsily written. In spite of this handicap, one of these, George Lillo's *The London Merchant* (1731), suggested the potentiality of this type of play and was indeed influential on German dramatic theory and practice. However, no systematic attempt was made in England to develop what Lillo had begun, and tragedy very nearly became extinct.

In contrast, a strong revival of comedy can be seen in the period now under consideration. A second wave of the comedy of manners was begun by Southerne in 1691 with his brilliant psychological study, *The Wives Excuse.* Two years later, the Irish dramatist William Congreve presented his first success, *The Old Batchelor,* and a new though brief rejuvenation of comic form was under way. Within a few years, Vanbrugh, Burnaby, and Farquhar added their contributions. Historically, the most striking aspect of their work was their originality. Traditional comedy, before and after this group, presented the formula of boy-meets-girl, boy-wins-girl. The comedies of this short period, say 1691 to 1707, deal with marital incompatibility, and in most of the plays either the hero or the heroine or both are already married as the play begins. If the main characters are not married, as with Mirabell and Millamant, we encounter a long proviso scene dealing with the causes of marital discord. A variant approach, found in Lord Lansdowne's comedy *The She Gallants* (1695), is the inclusion of a symposium on the problem of marital disharmony. (The play is so self-conscious that one at first suspects it was funded by the Arts Council.) There is no doubt that the playwrights were fully aware of the novelty of their structure and their break with convention. In the last comedy of this group, *The Beaux Stratagem,* Farquhar several times quotes or paraphrases from Milton's second divorce tract. Oblique evidence of authorial awareness can be found in the comparison of Vanbrugh's plots. In *The Relapse* (1696), the heroine, Amanda, is a sweet, innocent, virtuous woman, beyond the reach of the most passionate appeals of a would-be seducer. Her husband, Careless, is a confirmed woman-chaser. The point of the play is that he is incapable of reform. In *The Provok'd Wife* (1697), the husband, Sir John Brute, is a vulgar scoundrel, a vicious drunkard; his wife despises him and would like to cheat, save that she lacks the intestinal fortitude to commit adultery – virtue or morality are not her concern. In Vanbrugh's incompleted work *A Journey to London* (revised and finished later by Colley Cibber as *The Provoked Husband*), the male lead, Sir Francis Headpiece, is thoroughly honest and decent; his young wife is a huzzy who wants to go to London in the hope of getting sexual experiences. Vanbrugh's plan for ending the play was to have Sir Francis turn this rotten woman out of the house. The plays of this "Marriage Group" certainly deserve more attention.

Farce and burlesque again burgeoned. The most famous burlesque was the completely original ballad opera, *The Beggar's Opera* (1728). In it, John Gay achieves the irony peculiar to the Augustan age, in fact, so much so that some critics have erroneously called Swift the author. Originality also marks the lively experiments of Henry Fielding during his tenure as manager of the little theatre in the Haymarket. In *The Author's Farce* (1730), he attempted non-representational drama. His satire *Pasquin* (1736) enjoyed a sensational run. Fielding introduced footlights, offered two new plays on the same night, abandoned older drama, encouraged experimental work by young authors, employed the greatest care and pains to produce Lillo's tragedy of fate, *Fatal Curiosity* (1736), used actors in the audience, and invented an entirely original kind of dramatic burlesque in *The Tragedy of Tragedies* (1731). This experimental and innovative activity was completely ended by Sir Robert Walpole's interference in the Stage Licensing Act of 1737.

### 3. The Drama from 1737 to 1800

The drama experienced considerable change in the last half of the eighteenth century, though the differences may be more apparent to us than to audiences of the time. The age was dominated by comedy and comic opera, in spite of a large number of new tragedies. The plays become more thematic than before, and plot becomes increasingly important, leading to complex and involved structures by the end of the century in melodrama. Again, the audiences saw superior acting. Nevertheless, while some roles in new plays were designed for specific actors or actresses, this practice diminished in contrast to that of earlier periods, yielding to skilled ensemble acting. And in spite of some striking individual triumphs, the dramatists lost their previous pre-eminence of creating new dramatic forms, and were affected by foreign influences, notably the Italian comic opera, the French *comédie larmoyante,* and the lurid German melodramas of Kotzebue.

First, however, one should consider the altered conditions in the theatres for which the dramatists wrote. As a consequence of the restriction of legitimate drama in London to two theatres stipulated by the Stage Licensing Act of 1737, a considerable number of veteran players were available to the managers of the two remaining theatrical companies, Drury Lane and Covent Garden. Given a monopoly and a surplus of experienced actors, the managers preferred to drill, rehearse, and perfect their forthcoming productions of older works, especially after David Garrick became manager at Drury Lane, than to give up the proceeds of the third nights of the opening run to authors of new plays. A glance at the daily calendar in *The London Stage* will show how few new five-act plays appeared in the 1740's and 1750's. Meanwhile, partly from the sponsorship and financial backing of the "Ladies Shakespeare Club," a highly popular revival of Shakespeare's plays got under way. David Garrick soon learned that polished presentations of *Richard III, Hamlet, Romeo and Juliet,* and Jonson's *Every Man in His Humour,* alternated with later favorites, such as *The Beaux Stratagem* and *The Provok'd Wife,* would yield enormous financial rewards and avoid not only payments to authors but also disastrous failures at premieres. In this situation, it is not surprising that the best creative writers turned to writing novels, and English drama lost the high status it had maintained since the 1580's.

The players to sustain the roles were certainly available. At first there were Garrick, Spranger Barry, Kitty Clive, Peg Woffington, and Susannah Arne Cibber; later came J. P. Kemble, John Palmer, and Sarah Siddons. Numerous commentators called the cast for the premiere of *The School for Scandal* (1777) the best that had ever been assembled.

In time, new playwrights emerged. Their offerings in tragedy had little merit, but a number of popular comedies appeared, reflecting and refracting the mores of upper-middle-class Georgian society. Some of these comedies retained aspects of satiric analysis associated with Restoration drama, though a capacity for feeling becomes a test of individual value by the end of the play. Nevertheless, in portraying the idiosyncracies of the individual in society, most of the dramatists − from the talented to the mediocre − were what Stuart Tave has called "amiable humorists." Yet we must not forget that these playwrights were concerned with the problems of the current social world.

In older histories of English literature, these plays are written off as sentimental, with the implication that the audiences must have been naive to accept such simple stuff. This traditional estimate overlooks two important aspects of late eighteenth-century England: the cultural polish of the age and the concern with problem-solving. The reader needs to remember that the new elite which was coming into ascendancy early in the century (and which was the butt of the Tory satirists) was now in its second and third generation. For this new class, the brothers Adam designed and decorated the interiors of the houses, Thomas Chippendale and Thomas Sheraton made their chairs, Josiah Wedgwood their dinner ware, John Baskerville and William Caslin created the type for the books they read, and Joshua Reynolds, George Romney, Henry Raeburn, and Thomas Gainsborough painted their portraits. If these artifacts indicate a measure of elegance, why should the recipients lose their sophistication when they attended the theatre? Were not the plays an integral part of Georgian culture?

To illustrate the study of society in the drama of the period, I want to examine one play, Charles Macklin's highly popular comedy *The Man of the World* (1764). The author presents a nouveau riche Scot, Sir Pertinax Macsycophant, a recently created knight, firmly on the road to success. His grand plan is to marry his son, Egerton, into a noble family and obtain an estate. (Macsycophant has legally changed his son's name to get a small inheritance and to conceal his Scottish origin.) An heiress, Lady Rodolpha, is found, the daughter of land-poor Lord Lumbercourt, whose control over rotten boroughs provides him with two representatives in Parliament. Macsycophant supplies the money and enriches the noble lord, but Lumbercourt's lawyer delays the transaction, When the Scot discovers that this attorney wants to become an M.P., he quickly promises him the seat, with the result that the lawyers on both sides are working for the Scot. Meanwhile, Macsycophant sends his son out to attend levees of influential noblemen and expand his connections by flattering his way into their good graces. Egerton, just arrived from his course of studies at Oxford, refuses, whereupon the father denounces the Oxford tutor, Sidney, as "subversive." The irony here is delicious: Macsycophant had arranged for the best education for his son that money could buy, and Sidney had been dutifully transmitting to Egerton the newest ideas of the time – the revolutionary principles of the French Enlightenment, including the doctrine of the equality of mankind – and consequently really was subversive. In plotting this situation, Macklin was hardly less satiric than John Wilkes in his essays in the *North-Briton* on the Scottish invasion in the time of Lord Bute. George III was drawing upon the full powers of government to imprison and punish Wilkes, while the Lord Chamberlain refused for seventeen years to license *The Man of the World* for a stage performance.

Also, as I have indicated, there was a shift in the focus of interest in the ideas of the time, so that people were concerned with solving problems rather than raising them. In the seventeenth century, speaking broadly, one can say that the prime interest was in raising difficult questions. The authors of the heroic play showed the prince in agonized distress over the conflict between his private and personal interests and his duties as the ruler of a kingdom. The comic dramatists showed an irreconcilable clash between man's natural desires and the artificial conventions of the society in which he lived. In *The Country-Wife,* Lady Fidget wants to go to bed with any available man, but as the wife of a prominent London businessman, she has social constraints upon her behaviour. The consequences of truth-telling make up the contents of *The Plain-Dealer,* and the possible disadvantages arising from a liberal education afford matter for Shadwell's *The Squire of Alsatia* (1688). Southerne shows the impasse when a virtuous woman is married to a cowardly and inveterate woman-chaser, in *The Wives Excuse.* From these and other Restoration plays, we can observe that the playwrights were fond of dealing with discordant aspects of society. In the eighteenth century, however, the major thrust of the Enlightenment was towards the reform and solution of social ills, and the intellectuals wanted to see problems solved. In Richard Cumberland's *The West Indian* (1771), often called the prototype or model for late eighteenth-century comedy, the protagonist, Belcour, opens the play as a rake and a confirmed girl-chaser. After a number of adventures, Belcour is shown that he can become a useful member of society. In the penultimate speech of the play, Stockwell gives his verdict: "Yes, Belcour, I have watched you with a patient, but enquiring eye, and I have discovered through the veil of some irregularities, a heart beaming with benevolence, an animated nature, fallible indeed, but not incorrigible; and your election of this excellent young lady makes me glory in acknowledging you to be my son." There is no denial of the presence of evil: *Each One Has His Fault* (1792) Mrs. Inchbald announces as the title of her play; but intelligent and reasonable people can learn through experience.

Looking at the entire period, we can distinguish five relatively distinct varieties or types of drama: genteel comedy, humanitarian drama, musical comedy, farce, and tragedy. The works in the first category are those which deal with upper-middle-class society, from which they derive the nomenclature of "genteel." This was the term by which they were known at the time and it is a more accurate and hence more useful designation than the label of "sentimental comedy." The comic dramatists of this era were not trying to imitate *The Man of Mode,* nor should each of their works be measured against *The Way of the World* in order to assign a school grade, but should rather be studied in the context of literature and society of the Georgian period. Some, like Cumberland's *The West Indian,* place more stress on "feeling" and susceptibility to emotion than, say, Macklin's *The Man of the World.* The best known are the sparkling comedies of Sheridan (*The Rivals,* 1775, and *The School for Scandal*) and Goldsmith (*She Stoops to Conquer,* 1773), delightful plays which have held the stage since their premiere. A number of authors contributed at least one successful comedy of this sort. The earliest was Benjamin Hoadley's *The Suspicious Husband,* which opened at Drury Lane in 1747 and which was described at that time as the first good, full-length comedy in many years. The elder Colman's popular work, *The Clandestine Marriage* (1766), in which he was assisted by Garrick is an excellent example of genteel comedy, with its satire on social climbers and ridicule of fads in landscape gardening. Equally popular was *The Way to Keep Him* (1760), one of several comic treatments of marital incompatibility with which Arthur Murphy regaled theatre-goers. In addition to its long record of stage performances, this play was drawn upon for private theatricals possible more than any other drama of the time. Hugh Kelly's *False Delicacy* (1768), containing the criticism indicated by its title, was another lively, problem-solving comedy which enjoyed great popularity. A final example is Frederick Reynolds's *The Dramatist* (1789), in which the playwright Vapid upsets the villain's machinations by leaping up from concealment in a closet to spout the needed hemistitch to a line in an epilogue on which he had been straining his wits all day. All of these plays have been revived in modern times, and all contain considerable merit.

One entirely new species emerged toward the end of the century. It is known as "humanitarian drama," and the reasons for its failure as dramatic art are instructive. The chief practitioners were Thomas Holcroft, Richard Cumberland, and Elizabeth Inchbald. They were devoted to those basic principles of the European Enlightenment which Sir Pertinax Macsychophant had denounced as subversive. These playwrights were particularly interested in propagating the doctrines of the equality of mankind and the brotherhood of man. In the prologue to his chief stage success, *The Road to Ruin* (1792), Holcroft states that he is "Telling us that Frenchman, and Polishman, and every man is our brothers:/And that all men, ay, even poor Negro men, have a right to be free, one as well as another!" Cumberland even composed a play called *The Jew* (1794) for the explicit purpose of illustrating the concept of the brotherhood of man. In *Such Things Are* (1787), Mrs. Inchbald presented the prison reformer John Howard as a character in the play. In *Love's Frailties* (1794), Holcroft has one character say, "I WAS BRED TO THE MOST USELESS, AND OFTEN THE MOST WORTHLESS, OF ALL PROFESSIONS: THAT OF A GENTLEMAN." (Allardyce Nicoll points out that Holcroft had these words printed in capital letters.) Strong language indeed, yet there is not a play among this group of "humanitarian" dramas which has literary or dramatic merit. A look at some of these plays will show what went wrong. In *The Road to Ruin,* whose prologue insisted that every man is our brother, the villain, Silky, is a Jew. In *Duplicity* (1781), to the second edition of which Holcroft inserted a preface saying that he "would rather have the merit of driving one man from the gambling table, than of making a whole theatre merry," a person named Osborne manipulates Harry's finances to prevent him from being ruined by the Jews, and people from Somersetshire are presented as boobies. In *The Deserted Daughter* (1795), Holcroft offers a stereotyped comic butt in the Scot Donald. The melodramatic structure of Cumberland's *The Fashionable Lover* (1772) requires a villain, and the author provides a Scot for this purpose, along with a comic Jew, Naphtali. Mrs. Inchbald's plays are, as Allardyce Nicoll says, crammed with impossibilities, amazing discoveries, and heavy use of the "obscure birth" device as a plot solution. She also leans heavily upon stock characters. It is not a matter of lack of talent, for her plays include a number of valid and realistic touches. The trouble is that these playwrights were trying to put new wine into old bottles, unable to escape from the dominant theatrical conventions of the stock character – the stereotype. As a consequence, these plays do not generate dramatic conflict, and the use of stereotyped characters makes the message ludicrous.

It was the thesis of Bonamy Dobrée that high, satiric comedy emerged when a country had a highly cultured and stable society maintained over a considerable period of time, such as France in the age of Louis XIV. To a certain extent, conditions in late eighteenth-century London fit this formula, and hence the question may be asked why comedy did not develop beyond *The School for Scandal* and *The Clandestine Marriage.* The answer may seem facetious but it can be supported by stage history: high comedy lost out in competition with musical comedy. In the 1740's and 1750's, ballad opera had flourished, but these musical pieces were usually presented as the afterpiece to some longer work in the double-feature structure of London theatre programmes. Also, a few Italian comic operas had appeared from time to time. But this general situation was to change with the advent of Bickerstaff and

Dibdin. Peter Tasch shows, in his book on Isaac Bickerstaff, some amazing statistics abstracted from *The London Stage* to demonstrate the change. In 1755, the Covent Garden theatre was open on 184 nights. Tragedies and Shakespeare's history plays occupied 84 of these, comedy 85, and a musical production, either opera or oratorio, took up the remaining 15 performances. Ten years later, Covent Garden opened its doors for 189 performances, of which 81 were of musical comedies. The leader of this innovation was Isaac Bickerstaff, who found not only that English lyrics could be wed to music after the Italian manner but also the person who could perform the operation, the composer Charles Dibdin. Bickerstaff's first full-length musical comedy, *Love in a Village* (1762), was done with Thomas Arne, but Dibdin went on to compose or arrange the music for eight pieces by Bickerstaff, and to compose many more alone after Bickerstaff left the country. It will be noted that most of Dibdin's comic operas were based on French plays. General John Burgoyne supplied two more musical comedies, and showed full awareness that he was developing a new sub-genre by writing a defence of comic opera as a preface to his popular opus *The Lord of the Manor* (1780). The most popular of all of the many musical comedies was Sheridan's *The Duenna* (1775), a lively piece which achieved a run of seventy-five performances, the longest yet known on the London stage. Its success led to a nearly complete domination of musical comedy. The chief practitioner in the closing years of the century was John O'Keeffe, who composed about twenty comic operas, apart from his genuine comedy *Wild Oats*.

The particular satiric sting which we associate with Restoration comedy had gradually disappeared from the majority of five-act plays, as we have seen, but sharp ridicule re-appeared in an odd metamorphosis in the last half of the eighteenth century in the farces used as afterpieces in the double- and even triple-feature offerings of the London playhouses. Satire, invective, and mimicry all appear in the irregular pieces composed by Samuel Foote in his thirty-year residency at the Little Theatre in the Haymarket. Most of these plays or playlets were closely topical and directed at specific individuals, such as the attack on the Methodist evangelist George Whitefield in *The Minor* (1760). However, Foote achieved one artistic success in the mode of the great Augustan satirists – parodic satire – when he produced his farce *Piety in Pattens* (also known as *The Primitive Puppet-Shew*) in 1773. In it, as Samuel Bogorad writes in his recent edition of this farce, "Foote reduced to absurdity the sentimental vogue by portraying in Polly a housemaid who attempts to display the palpitatingly tender emotions of her betters." Richardson's *Pamela,* sentimental comedies, the new musical comedies, and the language of contemporary drama are all devastated in the opening lines of the piece: "In what a perilous State is a poor Maiden like me, beset every where, & no Friend to advise with. The Squire on one side, & the Butler on the other, no sooner as Mrs. Candy our Housekeeper says, have I escap'd the Silly of the Master, but I fall plump into the Cribbige of the Man." Successful as *Piety in Pattens* was on the stage, together with a tremendous amount of newspaper publicity, Foote never published his masterpiece. Two manuscripts, however, have been found in modern times, at the Folger and the Huntington libraries, and the farce has now been printed. Those who read it will realize that some textbook generalisations about the period will have to be altered.

In the 1760's, satiric farces flourished, led by Arthur Murphy, who exploited the comic possibilities of *l'idée fixe* in *The Apprentice* (1756) and *The Upholsterer* (1758) and skillfully built a harsh verbal duel from a dispute over a card game by a newly married couple in *Three Weeks after Marriage* (1764). The elder Colman contributed one lively piece in *Polly Honeycombe* (1760), and the actor Charles Macklin another in *Love A-la-Mode* (1759), with various other authors supplying satiric afterpieces until the end of the century. The last farce of the period to be a smash hit at the box office was Prince Hoare's *No Song, No Supper,* the music by Storace. The material in this musical farce came entirely from folklore, a sign of changing times.

The weakest drama of the period is found in the tragedies. The Augustan age did not lack a concept of tragedy, but an author who wished to present it would, for example, write it in prose in several volumes and call it *The Decline and Fall of the Roman Empire*. Not only were the playwrights unable to formulate a genuine tragedy but audiences preferred softened versions of Shakespeare's tragedies, such as Nahum Tate's emasculation of *King Lear*. Furthermore, the new serious plays which appeared were so completely under the domination of either French Classical tragedy or the new romantic stuff of Kotzebue and Schiller's *Die Rauber* that they merit only brief discussion. The most discussed new tragedy was John Home's *Douglas* (1756), looked on today as a most tedious play. Edward Moore made a feeble attempt to continue domestic tragedy in *The Gamester* (1753). The newer romantic mode is shown in Robert Jephson's *Braganza*. Actually, there was little room on the stage for tragedy, as the various forms or genres of drama at the end of the century tended to coalesce or merge, combining catastrophe, song, dance, comic stereotypes, and spectacle into the amorphous conglomeration called melodrama.

# READING LIST

## 1. Bibliographies, handbooks, etc.

Summers, Montague, *A Bibliography of the Restoration Drama*, 1934.

Harbage, Alfred B., *Annals of English Drama 975–1700*, 1940; revised edition, edited by Samuel Schoenbaum, 1964.

Woodward, Gertrude L., and James G. McManaway, *A Check-list of English Plays 1641–1700*, 1945.

Scouten, Arthur H., and others, editors, *The London Stage 1660–1800 · A Calendar of Plays, Entertainments, and Afterpieces*, 11 vols., 1960–68.

Stratman, Carl J., *Bibliography of English Printed Tragedy 1565–1900*, 1966.

Arnott, J. F., and J. W. Robinson, *English Theatrical Literature 1559–1900*, 1970.

Stratman, Carl J., D. G. Spencer, and M. E. Devine, editors, *Restoration and Eighteenth-Century Theatre Research: A Bibliographical Guide 1900–1968*, 1971.

## 2. General histories

Genest, John, *Some Account of the English Stage, from the Restoration to 1830*, 10 vols., 1832.

Ward, A. W., *A History of English Dramatic Literature to the Death of Queen Anne*, 3 vols., 1899.

Nettleton, G. H., *English Drama of the Restoration and Eighteenth Century*, 1914.

Nicoll, Allardyce, *A History of the Restoration Drama 1660–1700*, 1923; *A History of Early Eighteenth-Century Drama 1700–1750*, 1923; *A History of Late Eighteenth-Century Drama 1750–1800*, 1927; revised edition, 3 vols., 1952.

Dobrée, Bonamy, *Restoration Comedy*, 1924; *Restoration Tragedy*, 1929.

Bateson, F. W., *English Comic Drama 1700–1750*, 1929.

Craik, T. W., general editor, *The Revels History of Drama in English: Volume V: 1660–1750*, by John Loftis, Richard Southern, Marion Jones, and Arthur H. Scouten, 1976; *Volume VI: 1750–1880*, by M. R. Booth, Richard Southern, F. and L. Marker, and Robertson Davies, 1975.

Hume, Robert, D., *The Development of English Drama in the Late Seventeenth Century*, 1976.

### 3. Topics, themes, short periods, etc.

Palmer, J., *The Comedy of Manners*, 1913.

Bernbaum, E., *The Drama of Sensibility 1696–1780*, 1915.

Krutch, Joseph Wood, *Comedy and Conscience after the Restoration*, 1924; revised edition, 1949.

Lynch, Kathleen, *The Social Mode of Restoration Comedy*, 1926.

Hotson, Leslie, *The Commonwealth and Restoration Stage*, 1928.

Green, C. C., *The Neo-Classic Theory of Tragedy in England During the Eighteenth Century*, 1934.

Nolte, Fred O., *The Early Middle-Class Drama 1696–1774*, 1935.

Green, F. C., *Minuet*, 1935.

Summers, Montague, *The Playhouse of Pepys*, 1935.

Prior, M. E., *The Language of Tragedy*, 1947.

Wilson, J. H., *The Restoration Court Wits*, 1948.

Smith, J. H., *The Gay Couple in Restoration Comedy*, 1948.

Fujimura, T. H., *The Restoration Comedy of Wit*, 1952.

Kronenberger, Louis, *The Thread of Laughter*, 1952.

Hughes, Leo, *A Century of English Farce*, 1956.

Sherbo, Arthur, *English Sentimental Drama*, 1957.

Holland, Norman N., *The First Modern Comedies · The Significance of Etherege, Wycherley, and Congreve*, 1959.

Loftis, John, *Comedy and Society from Congreve to Fielding*, 1959.

Waith, Eugene M., *The Herculean Hero*, 1962.

Knight, G. Wilson, *The Golden Labyrinth · A Study of English Drama*, 1962.

Singh, S., *The Theory of Drama in the Restoration Period*, 1963.

Brown, John Russell, and B. Harris, editors, *Restoration Theatre*, 1965.

Loftis, John, editor, *Restoration Drama: Modern Essays in Criticism*, 1966.

Miner, Earl, editor, *Restoration Dramatists: A Collection of Critical Essays*, 1966.

Rothstein, E., *Restoration Tragedy: Form and Process and Change*, 1967.

Muir, Kenneth, *The Comedy of Manners*, 1970.

Birdsall, V. O., *Wild Civility: The English Comic Spirit on the Restoration Stage*, 1970.

Loftis, John, *The Spanish Plays of Neoclassical England*, 1973.

### 4. Anthologies of primary works

*Bell's British Theatre*, 21 vols., 1776–81; supplement, 4 vols., 1785.

Inchbald, Mrs., editor, *British Theatre*, 25 vols., 1808; supplement, 7 vols., 1809.

Spingarn, J. E., editor, *Critical Essays of the Seventeenth Century*, 3 vols., 1908–09.

Summers, Montague, editor, *Restoration Comedies*, 1922.

Stevens, D. H., editor, *Types of English Drama*, 1923.

MacMillan, Dougald, and Howard Mumford Jones, editors, *Plays of the Restoration and 18th Century*, 1931.

Elson, J. J., editor, *The Wits* (interregnum drolls), 1932.

Nettleton, G. H., and Arthur E. Case, editors, *British Dramatists from Dryden to Sheridan*, 1939; revised edition, edited by G. W. Stone, 1975.

Hughes, Leo, and Arthur H. Scouten, editors, *Ten English Farces*, 1948.

Wilson, J. H., editor, *Six Restoration Plays*, 1959.

Spencer, Christopher, editor, *Five Restoration Adaptations of Shakespeare*, 1965.

Trussler, Simon, editor, *Burlesque Plays of the Eighteenth Century*, 1969.

Bevis, R. W., editor, *Eighteenth-Century Drama · Afterpieces*, 1970.

Rubsamen, W. H., editor, *The Ballad Opera*, 28 vols., 1974.

Sutherland, James, editor, *Restoration Tragedies*, 1977.

**BANKS, John.** English. Very little is known about his life: flourished 1677–96. Studied law; a member of the society of the New Inn.

PUBLICATIONS

Plays

    *The Rival Kings; or, The Loves of Oroondates and Statira* (produced 1677). 1677.
    *The Destruction of Troy* (produced 1678). 1679.
    *The Unhappy Favourite; or, The Earl of Essex* (produced 1681). 1682; edited by James
       Sutherland, in *Restoration Tragedies*, 1976.
    *Virtue Betrayed; or, Anna Bullen* (produced 1682). 1682.
    *The Island Queens; or, The Death of Mary, Queen of Scotland.* 1684; revised version,
       as *The Albion Queens* (produced 1704), 1704.
    *The Innocent Usurper; or, The Death of the Lady Jane Gray.* 1694.
    *Cyrus the Great; or, The Tragedy of Love* (produced 1695). 1696.

Reading List: Introduction by Thomas M. H. Blair to *The Unhappy Favourite*, 1939; *Banks: Eine Studie* by Hans Hochuli, 1952.

\*    \*    \*

John Banks is certainly one of the weakest playwrights in the long history of English drama and he was not even considered a poet by his later contemporaries. Yet he was responsible for a major change in tragedy and he was an innovator in turning to recent English history as subject matter for his most popular plays. In making a woman the central character, he brought about a sweeping change in the nature of English tragedy. The prevailing pattern of earlier drama showed the fall of a strong hero – Faustus, Richard III, Bussy d'Ambois, Lear, Coriolanus; the current mode of the heroic play had its Almanzors and Montezumas; Banks offered, instead, a heroine in distress. In fact, in two of his most popular plays both the heroine and the villain are women. Critics sneered and termed his plays "she-tragedies," but the dramatists fell in line – Otway, Southerne, Congreve, and especially Nicholas Rowe – to follow this major shift in tragic structure.

A basic characteristic of the contemporary heroic drama was its distant setting, and the action was often set at a remote time. Banks showed considerable initiative in choosing his material for historical events in the lifetime of Queen Elizabeth I. Deficient as he was in attempting verse, he had no difficulty in recognizing tragic episodes from history: the plight of Anne Boleyn, the ordeal of decision by Queen Elizabeth on the Earl of Essex and Mary, Queen of Scots. Some of these events were scarcely a century old, it will be recalled. This fact, together with the native setting, probably created a strong sense of realism for Restoration audiences, and provided a striking contrast to the purposeful artificiality of the heroic drama. The subject matter of "real" versus "usurping" rulers and the deposition and execution of queens led of course to many of the plays being banned from the stage.

—Arthur H. Scouten

**BEHN, Aphra (Johnson).** English. Born, probably in Harbledown, Kent, baptized 14 December 1640. Probably married a Mr. Behn c. 1664 (died before 1666). Lived in Surinam, Dutch Guiana, c. 1663–64; employed by the English as a spy in Antwerp in 1666; imprisoned for debt in late 1660's; professional writer. *Died 16 April 1689.*

PUBLICATIONS

Collections

*Works,* edited by Montague Summers.   6 vols., 1915.
*Selected Writings,* edited by Robert Phelps.   1950.

Plays

*The Forced Marriage; or, The Jealous Bridegroom* (produced 1670).   1671.
*The Amorous Prince; or, The Curious Husband* (produced 1671).   1671.
*The Dutch Lover* (produced 1673).   1673.
*Abdelazar; or, The Moor's Revenge,* from the play *Lust's Dominion* (produced 1676).   1677.
*The Town Fop; or, Sir Timothy Tawdrey* (produced 1676).   1677.
*The Debauchee; or, The Credulous Cuckold,* from the play *A Mad Couple Well Matched* by Richard Brome (produced 1677).   1677.
*The Rover; or, The Banished Cavaliers* (produced 1677).   1677; edited by Frederick M. Link, 1967.
*Sir Patient Fancy* (produced 1678).   1678.
*The Feigned Courtesans; or, A Night's Intrigue* (produced 1679).   1679.
*The Young King; or, The Mistake* (produced 1679).   1683.
*The Revenge; or, A Match in Newgate,* from the play *The Dutch Courtesan* by Marston (produced 1680).   1680.
*The Second Part of The Rover* (produced 1681).   1681.
*The Roundheads; or, The Good Old Cause,* from the play *The Rump* by John Tatham (produced 1681).   1682.
*The False Count; or, A New Way to Play an Old Game* (produced 1681).   1682.
*The City Heiress; or, Sir Timothy Treat-All,* from the play *A Mad World, My Masters* by Middleton (produced 1682).   1682.
*The Lucky Chance; or, An Alderman's Bargain* (produced 1686).   1687; edited by A. Norman Jeffares, in *Restoration Comedy,* 1974.
*The Emperor of the Moon* (produced 1687).   1687; edited by Leo Hughes and Arthur H. Scouten, in *Ten English Farces,* 1948.
*The Widow Ranter; or, The History of Bacon in Virginia* (produced 1689).   1690.
*The Younger Brother; or, The Amorous Jilt* (produced 1696).   1696.

Fiction

*Love Letters Between A Nobleman and His Sister.*   3 vols., 1683–87.
*The Fair Jilt; or, The History of Prince Tarquin and Miranda.*   1688.
*Oroonoko; or, The Royal Slave.*   1688.
*The History of the Nun; or, The Fair Vow-Breaker.*   1689.
*The Lucky Mistake.*   1689.

*Histories and Novels.*   1696; revised edition, 1697, 1700.


Verse

*Poems upon Several Occasions, with a Voyage to the Island of Love.*   1684.
*A Pindaric on the Death of Our Late Sovereign.*   1685.
*A Pindaric Poem on the Happy Coronation of His Sacred Majesty James II and His Illustrious Consort Queen Mary.*   1685.
*A Poem to Catherine, Queen Dowager.*   1685.
*To Christopher, Duke of Albemarle, on His Voyage to Jamaica: A Pindaric.*   1687.
*To the Memory of George, Duke of Buckingham.*   1687.
*A Poem to Sir Roger L'Estrange.*   1688.
*A Congratulatory Poem to Her Majesty.*   1688.
*A Congratulatory Poem to the King's Most Sacred Majesty.*   1688.
*To Poet Bavius.*   1688.
*Lycidus; or, The Lover in Fashion, Together with a Miscellany of New Poems by Several Hands,* with others.   1688.
*A Congratulatory Poem to Her Sacred Majesty Queen Mary, upon Her Arrival in England.*   1689.
*A Pindaric Poem to the Rev. Dr. [Thomas] Burnet.*   1689.


Other

Editor, *Convent Garden Drollery.*   1672; edited by G. Thorn-Drury, 1928.
Editor, *Miscellany, Being a Collection of Poems by Several Hands* (includes Behn's translation of La Rochefoucauld).   1685.

Translator, *La Montre; or, The Lover's Watch,* by Balthasar de Bonnecorse.   1686.
Translator, *The Fatal Beauty of Agnes de Castro,* by J. B. de Brillac.   1688.
Translator, *A Discovery of New Worlds,* by Fontennelle.   1688; as *The Theory of New Worlds,* 1700.
Translator, *The History of Oracles, and the Cheats of the Pagan Priests,* by Fontennelle.   1688.
Translator, with others, *Cowley's Six Books of Plants.*   1689.


Reading List: *Behn* by V. Sackville-West, 1927; *The Incomparable Aphra* by George Woodcock, 1948; *New Light on Behn* by W. J. Cameron, 1961; *Behn* by Frederick M. Link, 1968 (includes bibliography); *The Passionate Shepherdess: Behn* by Maureen Duffy, 1977.

\*　　\*　　\*

Aphra Behn began her literary career as a dramatist. Her early plays are undistinguished imitations of the romantic tragi-comedy deriving from Beaumont and Fletcher; *Abdelazar,* for instance, is a successful but conventional tragedy of blood and lust. Her first good play is *The Town Fop,* a racy London comedy combining complex intrigue, farce, and expert dialogue. This formula, often augmented by a pair of witty lovers, she repeats in later plays like *The Rover, Sir Patient Fancy, The Feigned Courtesans, The Second Part of The Rover,* and *The Lucky Chance. The False Count* is a romantic farce in the traditional manner; *The Emperor of the Moon* a fine farce in the new *commedia dell' arte* style. *The Roundheads* is clumsy Tory propaganda, but Behn's other political play, *The City Heiress,* is coherent and witty enough to rank with her best work. Two plays were produced posthumously; three others are usually attributed to her, *The Revenge* with near certainty.

Behn's comedies are action-focused. At their best, they show sure craft, an accurate ear for speech rhythms, considerable wit, and mastery of stagecraft. Most of them borrow from earlier European or English sources; a play wholly original, like *The Feigned Courtesans*, is unusual. Some works, like *The Lucky Chance*, make minor use of sources. Others, like *Sir Patient Fancy*, *The City Heiress*, and *The Emperor of the Moon*, borrow both plot suggestions and the outline of characters. *The Town Fop* and *The Rover* are among Behn's adaptations of earlier plays which are in every case better than the originals. What she borrows she makes her own; plot ideas may come from Killigrew or Molière, but dialogue, pace, organization, most detail, and stagecraft are nearly always original. Her themes sometimes go beyond the conventional, especially in her emphasis on mature relationships between the sexes and on the evils of marriages made for money instead of love, and many of her characters (Hellena in *The Rover*, for example) have a vitality that transcends the stereotypes of the period.

Behn's poetry is occasional. The elegies and panegyrics are inconsequential and often clumsy; the prologues, epilogues, and songs for the plays are generally successful and often excellent. Several forgettable translations of French and Latin works belong to her later years when she was desperate for money; even so, her version of La Rochefoucauld is better than one might expect. Her short fiction has been overrated. *The Fair Jilt*, a study of the *femme fatale*, and *The Wandering Beauty*, a pastoral fairy tale, are worth reading, but *Oroonoko*, which contrasts the nobility of a savage with the baseness of supposedly civilized Englishmen in Surinam, is the only piece comparable to her best comedies. The majority of these were stage successes; indeed, *The Rover* and *The Emperor of the Moon* survived nearly a century. Taken together, they rank Aphra Behn with Dryden, Etherege, Wycherley, and Shadwell among the comic dramatists of her day – no mean achievement for the first Englishwoman to make her living by her pen.

—Frederick M. Link

---

**BICKERSTAFF, Isaac.** Irish.  Born in Dublin, 26 September 1733. Soldier: Page to Lord Chesterfield, Lord Lieutenant of Ireland, 1745; commissioned Ensign in the Fifth Regiment of Foot, 1745, and 2nd Lieutenant, 1746 until he resigned, 1755; 2nd Lieutenant, 91st Company, Plymouth Marine Corps, 1758–63. Wrote for the stage, 1756–71; fled England to avoid arrest as a homosexual, 1772, and spent the remainder of his life in exile abroad. *Died c. 1808.*

PUBLICATIONS

Plays

    *Thomas and Sally; or, The Sailor's Return*, music by Thomas Arne (produced 1760).  1761; revised edition, 1780.
    *Judith* (oratorio), music by Thomas Arne (produced 1761).  1761.
    *Love in a Village*, music by Thomas Arne and others (produced 1762).  1763.
    *The Maid of the Mill*, music by Samuel Arnold and others (produced 1765).  1765.

*Daphne and Amintor,* from a work by Saint-Foix (produced 1765).    1765.

*The Plain Dealer,* from the play by Wycherley (produced 1765).    1766.

*Love in the City,* music by Charles Dibdin and others (produced 1767).    1767;
shortened version, as *The Romp* (produced 1774), 1786.

*Lionel and Clarissa,* music by Charles Dibdin (produced 1768).    1768; revised version,
as *The School for Fathers* (produced 1770), 1770.

*The Absent Man* (produced 1768).    1768.

*The Padlock,* music by Charles Dibdin (produced 1768).    1768.

*The Royal Garland,* music by Samuel Arnold (produced 1768).    1768.

*Queen Mab* (cantata), music by Charles Dibdin (produced 1768).    1768.

*The Hypocrite,* from the play *The Non-Juror* by Cibber (produced 1768).    1769.

*Doctor Last in His Chariot,* from a play by Molière (produced 1769).    1769.

*The Captive,* music by Charles Dibdin, from the play *Don Sebastian* by Dryden
(produced 1769).    1769.

*The Ephesian Matron; or, The Widow's Tears,* music by Charles Dibdin (produced
1769).    1769.

*Tis Well It's No Worse,* from a play by Calderón (produced 1770).    1770.

*The Recruiting Serjeant,* music by Charles Dibdin (produced 1770).    1770.

*He Would If He Could; or, An Old Fool Worse Than Any,* music by Charles Dibdin, from
a play by G. A. Federico (as *The Maid the Mistress,* produced 1770; as *He Would If He
Could,* produced 1771).    1771.

*The Sultan; or, A Peep into the Seraglio,* from a play by C. S. Favart, music by Charles
Dibdin and others (produced 1775).    1780.


Fiction

*The Life and Adventures of Ambrose Gwinnet.*    1768.


Verse

*Leucothoë: A Dramatic Poem.*    1756.


Reading List: *The Dramatic Cobbler: The Life and Works of Bickerstaff* by Peter A. Tasch,
1971; *English Theatre Music in the Eighteenth Century* by Roger Fiske, 1973.

*      *      *

Between 1760 and 1772, Isaac Bickerstaff was the dramatist primarily responsible for
originating English comic opera and making it fashionably popular. His plots were not new –
he adapted and borrowed from English and French plays more than he ever acknowledged –
but he paired music, much of it by continental composers, and only some of it commissioned
for his operas, with often witty and always singable lyrics.

*Love in a Village* is by critical assent the first English comic opera and the most popular in
the eighteenth century. Thomas Arne composed the music specifically for five of the forty-
two songs and used thirteen of his earlier melodies. Bickerstaff borrowed from Wycherley's
*The Gentleman's Dancing Master* and plundered Charles Johnson's *The Village Opera.*
Despite harsh criticism of his plagiarism, the comic opera was an overwhelming success (37
performances at Covent Garden during its first season). Bickerstaff repeated his success with
*The Maid of the Mill* in which Charles Dibdin, who became his composer two years later,
played the comic role of Ralph.

As successful as Bickerstaff and Dibdin were to be, their first superb effort, *Love in the City,* failed because its satire was too apposite for the London audience. Profiting from their mistake, they returned to pastoral plots for their next comic opera, *Lionel and Clarissa*. In the four comic operas which Bickerstaff wrote during the 1760's for Covent Garden, he developed the form of musical comedy which lasted until the time of Gilbert and Sullivan a hundred years later.

Unable to compete with Covent Garden, Garrick hired Bickerstaff and Dibdin, but their only full-length opera for Drury Lane was their revised *Lionel and Clarissa*, *School for Fathers*. However, Bickerstaff did write the musical farce, *The Padlock*, with Dibdin's music; and Dibdin played the comic servant Mungo in blackface – the first such occurrence on the London stage. Bickerstaff also adapted comedies like Wycherley's *The Plain Dealer* for Garrick. Although his most popular comedy, *The Hypocrite*, was based on Cibber's *Non-Juror*, Bickerstaff's character Maw-worm was original and kept the play alive well into the nineteenth century.

Bickerstaff's and Dibdin's most interesting musical works were two serenatas for Ranelagh House: *The Ephesian Matron* and *The Recruiting Serjeant*. These short Italianate light operas (similar in style to *La Serva Padrona*) might have led the two men to new musical dramatic forms, but in 1772 Bickerstaff's career ended when he fled to France to avoid arrest as a homosexual. Despite his short career, Bickerstaff is important to English drama because to it he contributed comic opera.

—Peter A. Tasch

---

**BOYLE, Roger;** Baron Broghill; 1st Earl of Orrery.    Irish.    Born in Lismore, 25 April 1621. Educated at Trinity College, Dublin; may have studied at Oxford University. Married Lady Margaret Howard in 1641; two sons and five daughters. Travelled in France and Italy for several years after leaving university, then went to England, and commanded the Earl of Northumberland's troops in the Scottish expedition; returned home to Ireland at the time of the rebellion, 1641: under the Earl of Cork took part in the defence of Lismore, and held a command at the battle of Liscarrol, 1642; served under the parliamentarians, 1647–48, but continued to support the Royalist, and later the Restoration, cause, until offered a general's command by Cromwell in the war against the Irish, 1650; after the defeat of the Irish appointed Governor of Munster, and given control of various estates in Ireland, including Blarney Castle; served the Commonwealth government as Member of Parliament for Cork, 1654, and for Edinburgh, 1656, as Lord President of the Council, 1656, as a Member of the House of Lords, 1657, and as one of Cromwell's special council; after death of Cromwell concluded that Richard Cromwell's attempts to consolidate the government were hopeless: obtained command of Munster, and with Sir Charles Coote, secured Ireland for Charles II; served as Lord President of Munster until 1668; appointed a Lord Justice of Ireland, 1660; Member of Parliament for Arundel, 1661; impeached by the House of Commons for taxing without the king's authority, 1668, which proceedings were stopped by the King's proroguing Parliament. Created Baron Broghill, 1627; Earl of Orrery, 1660. *Died 16 October 1679.*

PUBLICATIONS

Collections

*Dramatic Works,* edited by William S. Clark, II.    2 vols., 1937.

Plays

*The General* (as *Altamire*, produced 1662; as *The General*, produced 1664).   Edited by
J. O. Halliwell, 1853.
*Henry the Fifth* (produced 1664).   With *Mustapha*, 1668.
*Mustapha, Son of Solyman the Magnificent* (produced 1665).   With *Henry the Fifth*,
1668; edited by Bonamy Dobrée, in *Five Heroic Plays*, 1960.
*The Black Prince* (produced 1667).   In *Two New Tragedies*, 1669.
*Tryphon* (produced 1668).   In *Two New Tragedies*, 1669.
*Guzman* (produced 1669).   1693.
*Mr. Anthony* (produced 1669).   1690.
*Herod the Great*, in *Six Plays*.   1694.
*King Saul*.   1703.
*Zoroastres*, in *Dramatic Works*.   1937.

Fiction

*Parthenissa*.   6 vols., 1654–69.
*English Adventures*.   1676.
*The Martyrdom of Theodora and Didymus*.   1687.

Verse

*Poems on Most of the Festivals of the Church*.   1681.

Other

*A Treatise of the Art of War*.   1677.
*A Collection of the State Letters*.   1742.

Reading List: "An Unheroic Dramatist" by Graham Greene, in *The Lost Childhood and
Other Essays*, 1951; *Boyle* by Kathleen M. Lynch, 1965.

\*      \*      \*

Despite the opinion of Graham Greene – "Roger Boyle ... is one of the great bores of
literature" – the First Earl of Orrery remains a fascinating representative of Cavalier culture.
Nobleman, statesman, servant of the Stuart kings and of Cromwell, he also found time to
pursue a career as a man of letters. His plays, which include the first important attempts to
introduce rhymed heroic tragedy on the English stage, were admired by Dryden and
Davenant, and retained some popularity after the Restoration.
His contemporaries also knew him as the author of a work which has proved less
accessible to posterity – *Parthenissa*, one of the earliest and best English experiments with
long heroic romance in the manner of such French salon-writers as La Calprenède and the de
Scudérys. Orrery points out in his Preface that the book is a deliberate amalgam of history
and fiction, real and imaginary people, because "Historyes are for the most Part but mixt
Romances, and yet the Pure Romance Part, may be as Instructive as, if not more than, the
Historicall." Like its French models, *Parthenissa* interlaces pseudo-philosophical dialogues on
Platonic love and honour with descriptions of action – the pageantry of tournaments, and
battles on land and sea. It is structured around the intersecting stories of four pairs of high-

born lovers, of whom Parthenissa and Artabanes are the most important. The couples assemble at the Temple of Hierophanus in Syria to consult the oracle, and there exchange tales of trials in love and friendship, and hazards in war, in a prose which, though sometimes florid, often has a pleasing dignity and serenity. Orrery's aim was to bring all of his lovers to felicity, but the romance remained unfinished, and only one of the stories is resolved.

—J. C. Hilson

BROOKE, Henry.   Irish.   Born in Rantavan, County Cavan, c. 1703. Educated at Trinity College, Dublin, 1720; The Temple, London. Married his cousin Catherine Meares; 22 children. From c. 1725 divided his time between London and Dublin; became involved in English politics: because of difficulties caused by his championing the Prince of Wales against George II returned to Dublin and settled there, 1740: appointed Barrack-Master, Dublin, c. 1745; in later years suffered from mental debility. *Died 10 October 1783.*

PUBLICATIONS

Collections

*Poetical Works,* edited by Charlotte Brooke.   4 vols., 1792.

Plays

*Gustavus Vasa, The Deliverer of His Country* (as *The Patriot,* produced 1744; as *Gustavus Vasa,* produced 1805).   1739.
*The Female Officer* (produced 1740).   In *A Collection of Plays and Poems,* 1778.
*The Earl of Westmorland* (as *The Betrayer of His Country,* produced 1742; as *Injured Honour,* produced 1754).   In *A Collection of Plays and Poems,* 1778.
*The Triumph of Hibernia,* music by Niccolo Pasquali (produced 1748).
*Little John and the Giants* (as *Jack the Giant Queller,* produced 1749).   In *A Collection of Plays and Poems,* 1778.
*The Earl of Essex* (produced 1750).   1761.
*The Victims of Love and Honour* (produced 1762).   In *A Collection of Plays and Poems,* 1778.

Fiction

*The Fool of Quality; or, The History of Henry, Earl of Moreland.*   5 vols., 1764–70; edited by E. A. Baker, 1902.
*Juliet Grenville; or, The History of the Human Heart.*   1774.

Verse

*Universal Beauty.*   1735.

*Constantia; or, The Man of Law's Tale,* in *The Canterbury Tales Modernised,* edited by George Ogle.   1741.

*Fables for the Female Sex,* with Edward Moore.   1744.

*New Fables.*   1749.

*A Description of the College Green Club: A Satire.*   1753.

*Redemption.*   1772.


Other

*The Farmer's Six Letters to the Protestants of Ireland.*   1745; as *Essays Against Popery,* 1750.

*The Secret History and Memoirs of the Barracks of Ireland.*   1745.

*A New Collection of Fairy Tales.*   1750.

*The Spirit of Party.*   2 vols., 1753–54.

*The Interests of Ireland Considered.*   1759.

*The Case of the Roman Catholics of Ireland.*   1760.

*Trial of the Cause of the Roman Catholics.*   1761.

*A Proposal for the Restoration of Public Wealth and Credit.*   1762(?).

*A Collection of Plays and Poems* (includes, besides the plays listed above, *The Vestal Virgin, The Marriage Contract, Montezuma, The Imposter, The Contending Brother, The Charitable Association, Cymbeline, Antony and Cleopatra*).   4 vols., 1778.


Translator, *Tasso's Jerusalem Delivered* (books 1–2).   1738.

Translator, *A New System of Fairy; or, A Collection of Fairy Tales,* by Comte de Caylus.   2 vols., 1750.


Reading List: *Brookiana: Anecdotes of Brooke* by C. H. Wilson, 2 vols., 1804; *Memoirs of Brooke* by Isaac D'Olier, 1816; *Brooke* by H. Wright, 1927.


\*      \*      \*


The eighteenth century so abounds in truly great novelists that excellent or eccentric second-raters are ignored. John Wesley hailed *The Fool of Quality* as "one of the most beautiful pictures that ever was drawn in the world; the strokes are so fine, the touches so easy, natural, and affecting, that I know not who can survey it with tearless eyes, unless he has a heart of stone." Now it may win only a notice in some learned discussion of William Law's *A Serious Call to the Devout and Holy Life* or of Shaftesbury's sentimental philosophy. In fact, Brooke's sentimental and discursive picaresque novel, with its variety, vivacity, and breeziness, ought to be linked with the "free fantasia" school of fiction in Sterne's wake, and with an eye to the influence of Rousseau.

Brooke's tragedy *Gustavus Vasa* (banned in London as revolutionary but produced in Dublin as *The Patriot*), is better know than *The Fool of Quality.* It deals with the Job-like tribulations of the Nordic giant who in the years following 1521 strove to unify and strengthen the kingdom of Sweden. Strindberg's play of the same name centers on the man himself; Brooke centers on the manipulations of the plot, and ends with fustian bombast. Brooke's *Earl of Essex* escaped the "bow-wow" attack of Dr. Johnson on *Gustavus Vasa,* but is inferior to it.

Brooke's verse is of interest for two reasons. "Conrade," purporting to be a fragment of old Celtic saga, fits into the poetic revival of Irish poetry exemplified by the Ossian controversy.

Pope is said to have assisted Brooke in *Universal Beauty*, and the poem was highly praised in its day. Bonamy Dobrée (in *English Literature in the Early Eighteenth Century*) says that Brooke "most nearly made a real poem out of science"; like Erasmus Darwin's *Temple of Love*, it repays investigation. Brooke was also a sincere and articulate political writer, especially on the Jacobite tendencies of the Irish Catholics and the notorious penal laws.

—Leonard R. N. Ashley

**BUCKINGHAM, 2nd Duke of; George Villiers.**   English.   Born in Westminster, London, 30 January 1628; succeeded to the dukedom, 1628; raised by King Charles I with his own children. Educated at Trinity College, Cambridge M.A. 1642. At the beginning of the Civil War joined the King at Oxford and served under Prince Rupert at the storming of Lichfield Close, 1643; later committed to the care of the Earl of Northumberland; sent on a Continental tour, lived in Florence and Rome; served under the Earl of Holland, in Surrey, during the second civil war, 1648; after defeat of the Royalists, escaped to France; appointed by Charles II a Member of the Order of the Garter, 1649, and Privy Councillor, 1650; appointed General of the Eastern Association of Forces, 1650, also commissioned to raise forces for the King on the Continent; Commander-in-Chief of the English royalists in Scotland, 1651; lands sequestered, 1651; accompanied Charles II on his expedition to England, quarrelled with the King, and returned to exile in Holland, 1651; returned to England, 1657; imprisoned in the Tower of London, 1658–59; served with the forces of Lord Fairfax, 1660. Married Mary Fairfax in 1657; later associated with the Countess of Shrewsbury, by whom he had a son. Recovered his estates at the Restoration; became gentleman of the king's bedchamber, 1660, and Privy Councillor, 1662; Lord Lieutenant of the West Riding of Yorkshire, 1661–67; briefly imprisoned and stripped of office for opposition to government policies, 1667; served as the King's principal minister in the "Cabal" administration, 1667–69; appointed master of the horse, 1668; replaced by Arlington in the King's confidence and kept ignorant of private negotiations with the French King, 1669, 1670; negotiated treaties with France for attack upon Holland, 1670, 1672; appointed Lieutenant General, 1673; quarrelled openly with Arlington, whom the King supported, 1673, and censured by Parliament for the French treaties, and deprived of his offices by the King, 1674; joined the Country Party, and thereafter acted as a leader of the opposition in the House of Lords, working for the establishment of a Whig parliament; admitted Freeman of the City of London, 1681; after the accession of James II abandoned public career and retired to Yorkshire. *Died 16 April 1687.*

PUBLICATIONS

Collections

   *Works,* edited by Tom Brown.   1704; revised edition, 2 vols., 1715.
   *Works,* edited by T. Percy.   1806(?).

Plays

   *The Chances,* from the play by Fletcher (produced 1667).   1682.

*The Rehearsal* (produced 1671).   1672; revised version, 1675; edited by D. E. L. Crane, 1976.

*The Militant Couple, The Belgic Hero Unmasked,* and *The Battle,* in *Works.*   1704.

*The Country Gentleman,* with Robert Howard, edited by Arthur H. Scouten and Robert D. Hume.   1976.


Other

*A Letter to Sir Thomas Osborn upon the Reading of a Book Called The Present Interest of England.*   1672.

*A Short Discourse upon the Reasonableness of Men's Having a Religion.*   1685.


Reading List: *Plays about the Theatre* by Dane F. Smith, 1936; *Great Villiers* by Hester W. Chapman, 1949; *The Burlesque Tradition in the English Theatre after 1660* by V. C. Clinton-Baddeley, 1952; *A Rake and His Times* by John H. Wilson, 1954; "*The Rehearsal*: A Study of Its Satirical Methods" by Peter Lewis, in *Durham University Journal,* March 1970.

*        *        *

Just as *Don Quixote* and *The Dunciad* have outlived the hack writing they parodied, so Buckingham's *The Rehearsal* survives as an eminently stageworthy play, while the heroic tragedies it burlesqued are studied more often for the theories justifying their form than for their intrinsic interest. *The Rehearsal* was Buckingham's single major contribution to the drama (though his adaptation of Fletcher's *The Chances* is still occasionally preferred to its original), for he was, as Dryden claimed in *Absalom and Achitophel,* "everything by starts, and nothing long," a man of curious vice, and considerable virtuosity.

Though first drafted in the mid-1660's, *The Rehearsal* did not reach the stage till 1671, by which time the heroic dramas of Davenant, Boyle, Dryden, Stapylton, and the Howards had successfully caught and held the public taste. In the following year, Dryden, recently created laureate, could still claim that heroic verse was "in possession of the stage," and that "very few tragedies, in this age, shall be received without it." That he himself shortly afterwards abandoned the form for good was in no small part due to the success of *The Rehearsal,* in which he is caricatured as the mock-dramatist Bayes.

The play anticipates many of the techniques perfected in the great age of burlesque, the early eighteenth century, in its rehearsal framework, and in its employment of "bathos," as re-defined by Pope. Its "plot" – the attempted usurpation of the two-seater throne of the Kingdom of Brentford – is bedecked with ludicrous imagery, absurd discoveries (a banquet appears out of a coffin), and contrived twists and turns in the action. Moreover, the framework permits Bayes to make a fool of himself in his own annotations to his play. Heroic drama could withstand charges of unreality (it was, after all, concerned with elevated behaviour): but Buckingham made it appear downright absurd, and so hastened its end.

—Simon Trussler

---

**BURGOYNE, John.**   English.   Born at Sutton Park, Bedfordshire, in 1722. Educated at Westminster School, London. Married Lady Charlotte Stanley in 1743 (died, 1776); had four children by Susan Caulfield. Soldier: cornet, 1740, lieutenant, 1741, and captain, 1744, in the 13th Light Dragoons; sold his commission and lived in France to escape his creditors,

1749–55; returned to England, obtained captaincy in the 11th Dragoons, 1756, and exchanged that commission for captaincy and lieutenant-colonelcy in the Coldstream Guards, 1758; served in expeditions to Cherbourg and St. Malo, 1758, 1759; devised schemes for creation of the King's Light Dragoons and Queen's Light Dragoons, 1759; sent to Portugal as Brigadier-General to assist the Portuguese against Spain: captured Valencia de Alcantara, 1762; Tory Member of Parliament for Midhurst, 1762–68, and for Preston, 1768–74; appointed Governor of Fort William, Scotland, 1769; Major-General, 1772; sent to the American colonies to reinforce General Gage's forces, 1774; during the Revolutionary War, Commander of the British attack of the United States from Canada: captured Ticonderoga and Fort Ward, and promoted to Lieutenant-General, then defeated by, and surrendered to, General Gates at Saratoga, 1777; on his return to England condemned for his actions by the House of Commons and the press, and deprived by the king of his commands and the governorship of Fort William; supported by the opposition and on return of Whigs to power appointed Commander-in-Chief in Ireland, 1782–83; thereafter devoted himself to writing. *Died 4 June 1792.*

PUBLICATIONS

Collections

*Dramatic and Poetical Works.*    2 vols., 1808.

Plays

*The Maid of the Oaks,* music by F. H. Barthelemon (produced 1774; revised version, produced 1774).    1774.
*The Lord of the Manor,* music by William Jackson, from a play by Jean-François Marmontel (produced 1780).    1781.
*The Heiress* (produced 1786).    1786.
*Richard Coeur de Lion,* music by Thomas Linley, from an opera by Michel Jean Sedaine, music by Grétry (produced 1786).    1786.

Other

*A Letter to His Constituents upon His Late Resignation.*    1779.
*A State of the Expedition from Canada.*    1780; supplement, 1780.
*Political and Military Episodes Derived from the Life and Correspondence,* by E. B. de Fonblanque.    1786.
*The Orderly Book from His Entry in the State of New York until His Surrender at Saratoga,* edited by E. B. O'Callaghan.    1860.

Reading List: *Gentleman Johnny Burgoyne* by Francis J. Hudleston, 1927; *The Man Who Lost America* by Paul Lewis, 1973.

\*        \*        \*

At Saratoga in 1777 General John Burgoyne lost an army. The fault was not his and the American commander who forced the surrender owed less to his own skill than to the complacency of the British Government and to the indolence of Burgoyne's superiors in North America. But Saratoga, the first battle-honour of the United States Army, spelt for Burgoyne the end of a long, gallant, and thoughtful career as a soldier. The fifteen years that were left to him Burgoyne used energetically and not often wisely. In Parliament as M.P. for Preston he was always ready to intervene on behalf of the Army and particularly of its private soldiers and non-commissioned officers, but his speeches were muddled and prolix and he was, not unnaturally, testy about his own military reputation. He wenched, he gambled, he roistered. But he also wrote, and the honours that had been denied him in his prime profession came his way eventually by way of the theatre.

His first dramatic piece, *The Maid of the Oaks* had been staged at Drury Lane before the American Revolution. It was damned by Horace Walpole (who damned almost everything that Burgoyne attempted whether in the Army, in Parliament, or for the stage), but David Garrick, better-qualified then Walpole to judge an entertainment, proclaimed it "a great success," and the play survived in the repertory for several months and, in book form, enjoyed a considerable vogue for many years. But it is in truth a heavy-handed and stylised piece, remarkable only for its mawkishness and portentous morality so utterly out of keeping with the author's personal inclinations and activities.

In *The Lord of the Manor* Burgoyne abandoned the ludicrously inappropriate pastoral idyll and took to the world he knew. Sergeant Sash, Corporal Dill, and Corporal Snip are caricatures only in the sense that they are exaggerations of reality, and Burgoyne understood the reality that is the British soldier. An eighteenth-century audience was never averse to a resounding platitude and Burgoyne gave them many to applaud, most of them from the lips of his *alter ego* hero, Trumore. *The Lord of the Manor* was written as a libretto, for the music of William Jackson of Exeter. Most of its faults are the faults of the operatic genre but they are as nothing when compared to the faults of Burgoyne's second attempt at opera, his adaptation of a serious French libretto, *Richard Coeur de Lion.*

*The Heiress* is a different matter. The plot is thin and moved forward in a flurry of coincidences. The characterisation is simplistic and is moulded almost entirely by the names of the participants (Lord Gayville; Mr. Rightly, the honest lawyer, and Mr. Alscrip, his devious colleague; Chignon, the prissy French hairdresser; the social climbers, Mr. and Mrs. Blandish) but the play has pace, the wit is sharp, and the social comment incisive.

With *The Heiress* Burgoyne made only £200 but he won the affection of the theatre-going public, of the critics, not only in England but also in France and Germany, and even of Horace Walpole: "Burgoyne's battles and speeches will be forgotten, but his delightful comedy *The Heiress* will continue the delight of the stage and one of the most pleasing domestic compositions."

—J. E. Morpurgo

---

**CAREY, Henry.** English. Born, probably in Yorkshire, c. 1687; believed by some scholars to have been the natural son of Henry Savile, Marquis of Halifax. Studied music with Olaus Linnert, Roseingrave, and Geminiani. Married in 1708; four children. Taught music in various boarding schools; settled in London, 1710; a member of Addison's circle; produced the magazine *The Records of Love*, 1710; wrote farces and songs for the London stage, 1715–39. *Died* (by suicide) *4 October 1743.*

PUBLICATIONS

Collections

*Poems*, edited by Frederick T. Wood.   1930.

Plays

*The Contrivances; or, More Ways Than One* (produced 1715).   1715; revised version, music by the author (produced 1729), 1729.
*Hanging and Marriage; or, The Dead-Man's Wedding* (produced 1722).   1722; revised version, as *Betty; or, The Country Bumpkins*, music by the author (produced 1732), songs published 1732.
*Amelia*, music by J. F. Lampe (produced 1732).   1732.
*Teraminta*, music by J. C. Smith (produced 1732).   1732.
*The Happy Nuptials*, music by the author (produced 1733).   Extracts in *Gentleman's Magazine*, November 1733; revised version, as *Britannia; or, The Royal Lovers* (produced 1734).
*The Tragedy of Chrononhotonthologos*, music by the author (produced 1734).   1734.
*The Honest Yorkshireman*, music by the author (produced 1735).   1736; pirated version, as *A Wonder*, 1735.
*The Dragon of Wantley*, music by J. F. Lampe (produced 1737).   1737.
*Margery; or, A Worse Plague Than the Dragon*, music by J. F. Lampe (produced 1738).   1738.
*Nancy; or, The Parting Lovers*, music by the author (produced 1739).   1739.
*Dramatic Works*.   1743.

Verse

*Poems on Several Occasions*.   1713; revised edition, 1720, 1729.
*Works* (songs and cantatas, with music by Carey).   1724; revised edition, 1726.
*Of Stage Tyrants: An Epistle*.   1735.
*The Musical Century* (songs).   2 vols., 1737; revised edition, 1740, 1743.
*An Ode to Mankind, Addressed to the Prince of Wales*.   1741.

Other

*A Learned Dissertation on Dumpling*.   1726.
*Pudding and Dumpling Burnt to Pot; or, A Complete Key to the Dissertation on Dumpling*.   1727.
*Cupid and Hymen: A Voyage to the Islands of Love and Matrimony*, with others.   1748.

Reading List: *English Comic Drama 1700–1750* by F. W. Bateson, 1929; *The Burlesque Tradition in the English Theatre after 1660* by V. C. Clinton-Baddeley, 1952; "Carey's *Chrononhotonthologos*: A Plea" by Samuel L. Macey, in *Lock Haven Review*, 1969; "Carey's *Chrononhotonthologos*" by Peter Lewis, in *Yearbook of English Studies*, 1974.

\*     \*     \*

Henry Carey thought himself a musician who wrote poetry for diversion. Posterity remembers him, if at all, for "Sally in Our Alley" and – debatably – for "God Save the King." Contemporaries knew him as a writer of popular songs, ballad operas, and burlesques. His poetic gift was meager; the classical imitations, moralistic and satiric pieces, and the heavier amatory verses are pedestrian at best. His only good poems are parodies like "Namby-Pamby," popular ballads like "Sally" and "The Town Spark and the Country Lass," and the lighter songs in his plays – "Oh, London Is a Dainty Place," from *The Honest Yorkshireman*, for example. Nor was Carey a well-trained musician. What he had was a knack for light rhymes and catchy tunes, and these together account for much of his success.

His first play, *The Contrivances*, was a smash hit after he turned if from farce to ballad opera; it was played nearly 200 times during the century. Carey also wrote both words and music for *Nancy; or, The Parting Lovers*, a short musical piece popular under several titles for decades. He supplied the music for a hit pantomime (*Harlequin Doctor Faustus*, 1723) and for a popular masque (*Cephalus and Procris*); much of the music for his ballad opera *The Honest Yorkshireman* is also original. *Amelia* and *Teraminta* show his interest in promoting English opera, but his librettos are flat and conventional; it was certainly J. F. Lampe's music which made *Amelia* a success.

Carey's real achievements, aside from *The Contrivances*, came late in his career. *Chrononhotonthologos* burlesques contemporary (and earlier) tragedy. No reader will easily forget the King of Queerumania and his court, or the opening lines of the play. Although not as directly parodic as *The Rehearsal*, it is delightful to read and stands comparison with *Tom Thumb*, its immediate predecessor. *The Dragon of Wantley*, a burlesque with music by Lampe, is even better, and was as popular for the rest of the century as *The Contrivances*. The plot, based on a laundered version of the ballad, is deliberately thin, and the burlesque of the Italian opera – evident in the music as well as the text – pointed and hilarious. So successful was the piece, indeed, that it nearly drove Italian opera off the English stage for a year or two. *Margery*, like most sequels, was less successful.

Carey is said to have heard his tunes everywhere he went. The modern reader is not so fortunate. No available edition of *The Dragon of Wantley*, for example, includes the music, yet it is as difficult to appreciate Carey's achievement without it as to judge *West Side Story* on its libretto. Like Isaac Bickerstaff and several other successful authors of the century, Carey remains largely inaccessible.

—Frederick M. Link

---

**CENTLIVRE, Susanna.** English. Born in or near Holbeach, Lincolnshire, 1669. Possibly married a nephew of Sir Stephen Fox, c. 1684, and an officer named Carroll, c. 1685; married Joseph Centlivre, principal cook to Queen Anne and George I, 1707. Actress in the provinces, often appearing in her own works, written under the name S. Carroll; devoted herself to writing from 1700; lived in London from 1712. *Died 1 December 1723.*

PUBLICATIONS

Collections

*Works.*   3 vols., 1760–61; as *Dramatic Works,* 1872.

Plays

*The Perjured Husband; or, The Adventures of Venice* (produced 1700).   1700.
*The Beau's Duel; or, A Soldier for the Ladies* (produced 1702).   1702.
*The Stolen Heiress; or, The Salamanca Doctor Outplotted* (as *The Heiress*, produced 1702).   1703.
*Love's Contrivance; or, Le Medecin Malgré Lui* (produced 1703).   1703.
*The Gamester,* from a play by J. F. Regnard (produced 1705).   1705.
*The Basset-Table* (produced 1705).   1706.
*Love at a Venture* (produced 1706?).   1706.
*The Platonic Lady* (produced 1706).   1707.
*The Busy Body* (produced 1709).   1709.
*The Man's Bewitched; or, The Devil to Do about Her* (produced 1709).   1710.
*A Bickerstaff's Burying; or, Work for the Upholders* (produced 1710).   1710; as *The Custom of the Country* (produced 1715).
*Mar-Plot; or, The Second Part of the Busy Body* (produced 1710).   1711.
*The Perplexed Lovers* (produced 1712).   1712.
*The Wonder! A Woman Keeps a Secret* (produced 1714).   1714.
*The Gotham Election.*   1715; as *The Humours of Election,* 1737.
*A Wife Well Managed* (produced 1724).   1715.
*The Cruel Gift; or, The Royal Resentment* (produced 1716).   1717.
*A Bold Stroke for a Wife* (produced 1718).   In *A Collection of Plays 3,* 1719; edited by Thalia Stathas, 1967.
*The Artifice* (produced 1722).   1723.

Verse

*A Trip to the Masquerade; or, A Journey to Somerset House.*   1713.
*A Poem to His Majesty upon His Accession to the Throne.*   1715.
*An Epistle to Mrs. Wallup, Now in the Train of the Princess of Wales.*   1715.
*A Woman's Case, in an Epistle to Charles Joye.*   1720.

Bibliography: "Some Uncollected Authors 14" by Jane E. Norton, in *Book Collector,* 1957.

Reading List: *The Celebrated Mrs. Centlivre* by John W. Bowyer, 1952.

*       *       *

Mrs. Centlivre wrote seventeen comedies, including three short farces, and strayed once or twice into tragedy. (Her poems are unimportant, orthodox complimentary or epistolary effusions for the most part.) Few of the plays were outright flops, and at least four enjoyed considerable success. The least merited popularity, perhaps, was that attached to *The Gamester,* a sentimental comedy rebuking the age for its addiction to gambling. A sequel, *The Basset-Table,* met with a less favourable reception, but it displays more vivacity in places, as in the scenes involving the uxorious City drugster Sago and his extravagantly flighty wife.

Throughout the eighteenth and nineteenth centuries, the dramatist's name was kept alive by two comedies which held the boards for decade after decade and which each totted up many hundreds of performances across the English-speaking world. Probably the better play is the earlier, entitled *The Busie Body,* constructed around the "sly, cowardly, inquisitive fellow" Marplot, who frustrates all the schemes he attempts to abet. This was a true acting part, and Theophilus Cibber, Henry Woodward, and Garrick all enjoyed great success in the role. Equally well-known was *The Wonder! A Woman Keeps a Secret,* which introduced some of Mrs. Centlivre's favourite Latin lovers – in this case melodramatic Portuguese grandees. Both the male and female leads provide fine opportunities for an accomplished player, and Garrick, Kemble, Mrs. Yates, and Susanna Cibber at various times all made a striking impact in the play.

Mrs. Centlivre's outstanding comedy is probably *A Bold Stroke for a Wife*, which traces the attempts of Colonel Fainwell to obtain the hand of Mrs. Lovely, a spirited heiress. The hero has to overcome the objections of four guardians, and he adopts a succession of disguises to deceive each of these well-marked "humour" characters – an antiquated beau, a foolish virtuoso, a grasping stock-jobber, and a sanctimonious Quaker. The play clearly exhibits the author's talent for lively dialogue, energetic stage business, and vivid portrayal of eccentric traits. It is worth adding that the unacted farce called *A Gotham Election* was an unlucky victim of political censorship. It is short but exceedingly amusing. The principal characters are conventional in outline, but nicely realised: for example, the amorous Squire Tickup, a Tory and seemingly a Jacobite into the bargain, who is opposed by the pompous Whig Sir Roger Trusty, a ready orator with a mouthful of high-minded party rhetoric always at his disposal. Around the gentry there are placed a wide range of rustic wiseacres, apparently foolish peasants with a vein of peasant shrewdness. As some of the names indicate – Shallow, Sly, Gabble – there is an echo of the Shakespearian clown in their speech, which is compounded of strange Mummerzet dialect and brutally direct colloquialisms. It is a pity that Susanna Centlivre did not get the opportunity to develop this vein of comedy; the play shows her capable of a realistic dramatic idiom rarely encountered on the eighteenth-century stage.

—Pat Rogers

---

**CIBBER, Colley.**   English.   Born in London, 6 November 1671. Educated at the Free School, Grantham, Lincolnshire, 1682–87. Joined the Earl of Devonshire's Volunteers, 1688, and remained in the service of the Earl of Devonshire, 1688–90. Married Katherine Shore in 1693; ten children. Actor in the Drury Lane Company, London, 1691–1706, and Adviser to the Manager after 1700, and Actor at the Haymarket, London, 1706 until the two theatres consolidated, 1708; Co-Owner/Manager of the Drury Lane Company, 1708–32; retired officially as an actor in 1733, but occasionally appeared on the stage until 1745. Poet Laureate, 1730 until his death. *Died 11 December 1757.*

PUBLICATIONS

Collections

*Dramatic Works.*   4 vols., 1760; 5 vols., 1777.
*Three Sentimental Comedies* (includes *Love's Last Shift, The Careless Husband, The Lady's Last Stake*), edited by Maureen Sullivan.   1973.

Plays

*Love's Last Shift; or, The Fool in Fashion* (produced 1696).   1696; in *Three Sentimental Comedies,* 1973.

*Woman's Wit; or, The Lady in Fashion* (produced 1697).   1697.

*Xerxes* (produced 1699).   1699.

*King Richard III*, from the play by Shakespeare (produced 1700).   1700; edited by Christopher Spencer, in *Five Restoration Adaptations of Shakespeare*, 1965.

*Love Makes a Man; or, The Fop's Fortune* (produced 1700).   1701.

*She Would and She Would Not; or, The Kind Imposter* (produced 1702).   1703.

*The Schoolboy; or, The Comical Rival*, from his own play *Woman's Wit* (produced 1703).   1707.

*The Careless Husband* (produced 1704).   1705; in *Three Sentimental Comedies*, 1973.

*Perolla and Izadora* (produced 1705).   1706.

*The Comical Lovers* (produced 1707).   1707; as *Marriage a la Mode* (produced 1707; as *Court Gallantry*, produced 1715).

*The Double Gallant; or, The Sick Lady's Cure* (produced 1707).   1707.

*The Lady's Last Stake; or, The Wife's Resentment* (produced 1707).   1708; in *Three Sentimental Comedies*, 1973.

*The Rival Fools* (produced 1709).   1709.

*The Rival Queens* (produced 1710).   1729; edited by William M. Peterson, 1965.

*Hob; or, The Country Wake*, from the play *The Country Wake* by Thomas Dogget (produced 1710).   1715.

*Ximena; or, The Heroic Daughter*, from a play by Corneille (produced 1712).   1719.

*Bulls and Bears* (produced 1715).

*Myrtillo*, music by J. C. Pepusch (produced 1715).   1715.

*Venus and Adonis*, music by J. C. Pepusch (produced 1715).   1715.

*The Non-Juror*, from a play by Molière (produced 1717).   1718.

*Plays.*   2 vols., 1721.

*The Refusal; or, The Ladies' Philosophy*, from a play by Molière (produced 1721).   1721.

*Caesar in Egypt* (produced 1724).   1724.

*The Provoked Husband; or, A Journey to London*, from a play by Vanbrugh (produced 1728).   1728; edited by Peter Dixon, 1975.

*Love in a Riddle* (produced 1729).   1729; shortened version, as *Damon and Phillida* (produced 1729), 1729; revised version, 1730.

*Polypheme*, from an opera by Paul Rolli, music by Nicholas Porpora (produced 1734).

*Dramatic Works.*   5 vols., 1736.

*Papal Tyranny in the Reign of King John*, from the play *King John* by Shakespeare (produced 1745).   1745.


Verse

*A Poem on the Death of Queen Mary.*   1695.

*The Sacred History of Arlus and Odolphus.*   1714.

*An Ode to His Majesty for the New Year.*   1731.

*An Ode for His Majesty's Birthday.*   1731.

*A Rhapsody upon the Marvellous Arising from the First Odes of Horace and Pindar.*   1751.

*Verses to the Memory of Mr. Pelham.*   1754.


Other

*An Apology for the Life of Mr. Colley Cibber, Comedian.*   1740; revised edition, 1750, 1756; edited by B. R. S. Fone, 1968.

*A Letter to Mr. Pope.*   1742; *Second Letter*, 1743; *Another Letter*, 1744.

*The Egoist; or, Colley upon Cibber.*   1743.
*The Character and Conduct of Cicero Considered.*   1747.
*The Lady's Lecture: A Theatrical Dialogue Between Sir Charles Easy and His Marriageable Daughter.*   1748.


Bibliography: by Leonard R. N. Ashley, in *Restoration and 18th-Century Theatre Research* 6, 1967.

Reading List: *Mr. Cibber of Drury Lane* by R. H. Barker, 1939; *Cibber* by Leonard R. N. Ashley, 1965; "Cibber's *Love's Last Shift* and Sentimental Comedy" by B. R. S. Fone, in *Restoration and Eighteenth Century Theatre Research 7,* May 1968.

*       *       *

Colley Cibber was a superb actor. In a career which lasted from 1691 (when he acted in a bit part in *Sir Anthony Love* by Thomas Southerne) till 1745 (when he starred in ten performances of his own *Papal Tyranny in the Reign of King John*) he created an army of cox-combs ("first in all foppery") and sneering villains (including his adaptation of *Richard III*). In all he played about 130 different parts. He was also one of the most important actor-managers in the history of the English stage. With others, he ran, for decades, the Theatre Royal in Drury Lane, and though he was sometimes criticized for his treatment of authors and inevitably made mistakes, he had a long and generally favorable influence on the stage.

He told the story of his public life in a brilliant autobiography, *An Apology for the Life of Mr. Colley Cibber, Comedian.* The real Cibber much resembles the striking, colored bust by Roubillac in London's National Portrait Gallery: a cheerful, shrewd, frank, ruddy face, the humorous expression of the rather thin lips suggesting that they might speak, probably with some self-satisfied vanity and with more than a little determination, some wisdom and more wit. The *Apology* covers 40 years of the London stage from the pen of a man who had a chief part in shaping its goals and achievements. The writer's style is conversational, his prejudices betrayed (or clearly stated), his friends defended, his enemies attacked, but this is a discussion of his professional, not his private, life. There is little here of Cibber the family man, the gambler, the *beau garçon.* His versatility and vitality dazzle us, his talent and tenacity win our admiration, and his very flaws and frailties endear him to us, for he is a true original (as Edward Young would say) even when he comes to us like an eastern potentate bedecked in light feathers.

Cibber aroused even more opposition than the *Apology* stimulated by gaining the appointment as Poet Laureate, though Gay was at pains to point out that a better man would not have accepted the job and a worse one could not have held it. Bad as he was, Cibber was, after all, the best Poet Laureate since Dryden, and it must be admitted that the odes which Joseph Knight recklessly called "the most contemptible things of literature" do not look so bad alongside those which Masefield (and more recent) laureates have perpetrated. Pope was biased but right to say Cibber's poetry was "prose on stilts," but Dr. Johnson was right too: "Colley Cibber, Sir, was by no means a blockhead."

Cibber's true worth was in his plays. His first play, *Love's Last Shift,* he wrote out of his "own raw uncultivated Head" and it was so good his enemies later swore it must have been stolen. It was a landmark in the history of English drama and launched the long vogue of sentimental comedy. For that (and the follow-up in this genre, *The Careless Husband*) Cibber's name must be featured in every history of the drama. Even his enemy John Dennis described it as having "a just Design, distinguished Characters, and a proper Dialogue." It's a good comedy. And *The Careless Husband* is a better one.

Cibber's tragedies are, on the whole, inferior to his comedies, though he has a deft hand with melodrama, and it must be noted that his version of *Richard III* replaced Shakespeare on the stage for about 125 years. The most famous of Cibber's *rifacimenti,* however, was

Molière's *Tartuffe* adapted as *The Non-Juror*; and the best-loved of Cibber's plays in his own time (second only to Shakespeare in popularity) was the comedy *The Provok'd Husband*. All of these are still worth attention.

Thus let us put Cibber down as Laureate and regret his odes, read his *Apology* and declare it too smug, praise his brilliant portrayals of the fop onstage and regret some of his private life offstage, criticize some of his comedic carpentry but recognize his occasional excellences and his undoubted place in the history of the drama, and accept Pope's diatribe in the *Dunciad* (which, after all, immortalized Cibber) while balancing it against Warburton's judicious estimate: "Cibber, with a great stock of levity, vanity, and affectation, had sense, and wit, and humor."

Leonard R. N. Ashley

---

**COLMAN, George, the Elder.**  English.  Born in Florence, Italy, where his father was envoy at court, in April 1732; returned to London, 1733. Educated at Westminster School, London, 1746–51; Christ Church, Oxford, matriculated 1751, B.A. 1755, M.A. 1758; Lincoln's Inn, London, 1755–57; called to the Bar, 1757. Married the actress Miss Ford (died, 1771); children include George Colman the Younger, *q.v.* Founding Editor, with Bonnell Thornton, *Connoisseur*, 1754–56; practised law on the Oxford circuit, 1759–64; left an income by his patron, the Earl of Bath, which allowed him to abandon the law, 1764; purchased one-quarter of the Covent Garden Theatre, 1767: Manager, 1767–74; retired to Bath; contributed to the *London Packet*, 1775; bought the Little Theatre, Haymarket, and managed it, 1777–89: paralysed by a stroke, 1785, and thereafter became increasingly feeble-minded; succeeded at the Haymarket by his son, 1789. *Died 14 August 1794.*

PUBLICATIONS

Plays

> *Polly Honeycombe: A Dramatic Novel* (produced 1760).  1760; edited by Richard Bevis, in *Eighteenth Century Drama: Afterpieces*, 1970.
> *The Jealous Wife*, from the novel *Tom Jones* by Fielding (produced 1761).  1761; edited by Allardyce Nicoll, 1925.
> *The Musical Lady* (produced 1762).  1762.
> *Philaster*, from the play by Beaumont and Fletcher (produced 1763).  1763.
> *The Deuce Is in Him* (produced 1763).  1763.
> *A Fairy Tale*, from the play *A Midsummer Night's Dream* by Shakespeare (produced 1763).  1763.
> *The Clandestine Marriage*, with David Garrick (produced 1766).  1766.
> *The English Merchant*, from a play by Voltaire (produced 1767).  1767.
> *The Oxonion in Town* (produced 1767).  1769.
> *King Lear*, from the play by Shakespeare (produced 1768).  1768.
> *Man and Wife; or, The Shakespeare Jubilee* (produced 1769).  1770.
> *The Portrait*, music by Samuel Arnold, from a play by Louis Anseaume, music by Grétry (produced 1770).  1770.

*Mother Skipton*, music by Samuel Arnold (produced 1770).    Songs published 1771.
*The Fairy Prince*, music by Thomas Arne, from the masque *Oberon* by Jonson (produced 1771).    1771.
*Comus*, music by Thomas Arne, from the masque by Milton (produced 1773).    1772.
*An Occasional Prelude* (produced 1772).    1776.
*Achilles in Petticoats*, music by Thomas Arne, from a work by John Gay (produced 1773).    1774.
*The Man of Business* (produced 1774).    1774.
*The Spleen; or, Islington Spa* (produced 1776).    1776.
*Epicoene; or, The Silent Woman*, from the play by Jonson (produced 1776).    1776.
*New Brooms! An Occasional Prelude*, with David Garrick (produced 1776).    1776.
*Polly*, from the play by John Gay (produced 1777).    1777.
*The Sheep Shearing*, music by Thomas Arne and others, from the play *A Winter's Tale* by Shakespeare (produced 1777).    1777.
*The Spanish Barber; or, The Fruitless Precaution*, music by Samuel Arnold, from a play by Beaumarchais (produced 1777).
*The Distressed Wife* (produced 1777).
*Dramatic Works*.    4 vols., 1777.
*The Female Chevalier*, from the play *The Artful Wife* by William Taverner (produced 1778).
*The Suicide* (produced 1778).
*Bonduca*, music by Samuel Arnold, from the play by Fletcher (produced 1778).    1778.
*The Separate Maintenance* (produced 1779).
*The Manager in Distress* (produced 1780).    1790.
*The Genius of Nonsense*, music by Samuel Arnold (produced 1780).    Songs published 1781.
*Preludio to The Beggar's Opera* (produced 1781).
*Harlequin Teague; or, The Giant's Causeway*, with John O'Keeffe (produced 1782).    Songs published 1782.
*Fatal Curiosity*, from the play by Lillo (produced 1782).    1783.
*The Election of the Managers* (produced 1784).
*Tit for Tat; or, The Mutual Deception*, from a work by Marivaux (produced 1786).    1788.
*Ut Pictura Poesis! or, The Enraged Musicians: A Musical Entertainment Founded on Hogarth*, music by Samuel Arnold (produced 1789).    1789.

Verse

*Two Odes*, with Robert Lloyd.    1760.
*Poems on Several Occasions*.    3 vols., 1787.

Other

*The Connoisseur*, with Bonnell Thornton.    4 vols., 1757.
*A Letter of Abuse to D—d G—k*.    1757.
*A True State of the Differences* (on Covent Garden Theatre).    1768.
*An Epistle to Dr. Kenrick*.    1768.
*T. Harris Dissected*.    1768.
*Prose on Several Occasions*.    3 vols., 1787.
*Some Particulars of the Life of George Colman, Written by Himself*.    1795.

Editor, with Bonnell Thornton, *Poems by Eminent Ladies*.    2 vols., 1755.

Editor, *The Works of Beaumont and Fletcher*.  10 vols., 1778.

Translator, *The Comedies of Terence*.  1765; revised edition, 1766.
Translator, *The Merchant*, in *Comedies of Plautus*.  1769.
Translator, *Epistola de Arte Poetica*, by Horace.  1783.

Reading List: *Memoirs of the Colman Family, Including Their Correspondence* by Richard B. Peake, 2 vols., 1841; *Colman the Elder* by Eugene R. Page, 1935; "Bickerstaff, Colman, and the Bourgeois Audience" by Peter A. Tasch, in *Restoration and 18th Century Theatre Research 9*, May 1970.

\*      \*      \*

The work of the many-faceted George Colman the Elder — lawyer, essayist, editor, translator, playwright, and theatre manager — is divisible into two phases: before and after 1764. In that year his uncle and patron, William Pulteney, Earl of Bath, died without fulfilling his nephew's great expectations, and this rude jolt sent a number of aftershocks through Colman's life and consciousness, as may be seen in his plays. Prior to 1764 he thought he was merely amusing himself at the bar and in the theatre until he could be made "easy," and his early dramatic efforts are commensurately light-hearted. *Polly Honeycombe*, "A Dramatick Novel of One Act," was an auspicious beginning; with strong acting by such comedians as Yates, King, and Miss Pope, who played the titular heroine on whom Sheridan modelled Lydia Languish, it pleased the town and gained a place in the repertory, giving Colman a quick reputation as a bright young man and a promising new comic voice. He followed this up the next season — with some editorial help from Garrick, according to tradition — by adapting *Tom Jones* for the stage as *The Jealous Wife*, his first full-length comedy and another success. *The Musical Lady* and *The Deuce Is in Him* kept his name before the public in the next two years without adding to his lustre or altering his "image"; both are two-act afterpieces.

What is notable about these first four plays — especially in view of his later work — is their general antipathy to sentiment, supposedly the prevailing taste at the time. *Polly* is a spirited attack on the sentimental novel (first cousin to the sentimental comedy), *The Deuce Is in Him* on one species of sentimentalist (the Tortuous Tester of Motives; compare Sheridan's Faulkland). *The Musical Lady*, supposedly culled from the overlong first draft of *Jealous Wife* but reminiscent of *Polly* in plot, is a thin wisp of manners satire. *The Jealous Wife* is mellower — as audiences expected a *main*piece to be — and has one rather sentimental reform scene, but is basically what Goldsmith later called a "laughing comedy." In these early plays Colman clearly feels that he is witty and amusing, and that he is free to choose his satiric targets without considering which of the drama's patrons might be in the line of fire.

The discovery that he was not to be a gentleman of leisure altered Colman's whole intellectual and emotional orientation from the free-wheeling to the careful; if he must "live to please," he "must please to live." After 1764 his tone changed rather suddenly from that of Foote to that of Garrick, and his mind kept reverting — understandably — to the simple but enormous difference between bourgeois and aristocrat. *The Clandestine Marriage*, co-authored with Garrick, tells the story of a poor young clerk who secretly marries his rich boss's daughter and then has to watch her being wooed by noblemen until the truth is revealed in act five. It is a very class-conscious play — at times almost an essay in sociology — that strikes a rough balance between laughter and sentiment, ridicule and sympathy, which made it quite popular with audiences of the time and gave Colman his greatest success. The 1975 London production survived by making Lord Ogleby, a comically senile rake probably created by Garrick, the centre of the play, leaving the distressed lovers to take care of themselves.

In 1767 Colman became manager of Covent Garden Theatre. His biggest coup in that position was producing *She Stoops to Conquer* in 1773 after Garrick had rejected it; otherwise his stewardship of Covent Garden (and later the Haymarket) was undistinguished. Presumably it was the demands of his managerial duties that made his subsequent efforts at dramatic authorship diffuse and relatively disappointing. He essayed most of the genres then current, but with a marked preference for the shorter, lighter and easier forms: farces, burlettas, spectacles, alterations. *The English Merchant*, adapted from Voltaire, is notable as Colman's most sentimental comedy, perhaps his only real one; both it and *The Man of Business* reveal his continuing preoccupation with the problems of the bourgeois, but their heaviness mars their gestures at social significance in a comic framework. Of his afterpieces in these years, *The Oxonian in Town* and *Man and Wife*, a gibe at Garrick's Shakespeare Jubilee in Stratford, have some entertainment value, while *New Brooms!* makes some interesting comments on theatrical taste and managerial dilemmas at the end of the Garrick era, when Sheridan took over Drury Lane.

Colman worked at a time when traditional tragedy and comedy were breaking down into new genres; perhaps he is best remembered as one of the first English writers of the *drame* or problem play. *The Man of Business* might be called a "comedy of fiscal responsibility," yet is also kin to the domestic tragedy of Lillo. It is filled with improving epigrams ("Regularity and punctuality are the life of business") and home questions ("What has a man of business to do with men of pleasure? Why is a young banker to live with young noblemen?") that the middle-class audience found piquant and relevant, and to which Colman himself could not have been oblivious. *The Suicide* returns to the theme of a young bourgeois toying with aristocratic vices, but in a bolder, darker, and more interesting way; it deserves more attention than it has ever received. Some of Colman's best writing is in the opening scene, of revellers returning at dawn to a London household just beginning to stir, and in the black comedy of the pseudo-suicide itself. His late play *The Separate Maintenance*, while less original, again shows Colman immersed in a contemporary social problem of genuine concern to his audience. Although he never decided exactly *what* point he wanted to make about the relationship between the bourgeoisie and the aristocracy, Colman's persistence in bringing living issues onto the London stage, at a time when most comedy was escapist, is significant on the eve of the French Revolution.

—R. W. Bevis

---

**COLMAN, George, the Younger.**    English.    Born in London, 21 October 1762; son of George Colman the Elder, *q.v.* Educated at a school in Marylebone, London, until 1771; Westminster School, London, 1772–79; Christ Church, Oxford, 1779–81; King's College, Aberdeen, 1781–82; Lincoln's Inn, London. Married 1) Clara Morris in 1784 (died); 2) the actress Mrs. Gibbs. Took over management of his father's Haymarket Theatre, 1789–1813 (purchased the Haymarket patent, 1794; disposed of all of his shares to his partner by 1820); appointed Lieutenant of the Yeoman of the Guard by George IV, 1820; Examiner of Plays, 1824 until his death. *Died 17 October 1836.*

PUBLICATIONS

Collections

   *Poetical Works.*    1840.
   *Broad Grins, My Night-Gown and Slippers, and Other Humorous Works,* edited by G. B.
      Buckstone.    1872.

## Plays

*The Female Dramatist,* from the novel *Roderick Random* by Smollett (produced 1782).
*Two to One,* music by Samuel Arnold (produced 1785).   1784.
*Turk and No Turk,* music by Samuel Arnold (produced 1785).   Songs published 1785.
*Inkle and Yarico,* music by Samuel Arnold (produced 1787).   1787.
*Ways and Means; or, A Trip to Dover* (produced 1788).   1788.
*The Battle of Hexham,* music by Samuel Arnold (produced 1789).   1790.
*The Surrender of Calais,* music by Samuel Arnold (produced 1791).   1792.
*Poor Old Haymarket; or, Two Sides of the Gutter* (produced 1792).   1792.
*The Mountaineers,* music by Samuel Arnold (produced 1793).   1794.
*New Hay at the Old Market* (produced 1795).   1795; revised version, as *Sylvester Daggerwood* (produced 1796), 1808.
*The Iron Chest,* music by Stephen Storace, from the novel *Caleb Williams* by William Godwin (produced 1796).   1796; edited by Michael R. Booth, in *Eighteenth Century Tragedy,* 1965.
*The Heir at Law* (produced 1797).   1800.
*Blue Beard; or, Female Curiosity! A Dramatic Romance,* music by Michael Kelly, from a play by Michel Jean Sedaine (produced 1798).   1798.
*Blue Devils,* from a play by Patrat (produced 1798).   1808.
*The Castle of Sorrento,* with Henry Heartwell, music by Thomas Attwood, from a French play (produced 1799).   1799.
*Feudal Times; or, The Banquet-Gallery,* music by Michael Kelly (produced 1799).   1799.
*The Review; or, The Wags of Windsor,* music by Samuel Arnold (produced 1800).   1801.
*The Poor Gentleman* (produced 1801).   1802.
*John Bull; or, An Englishman's Fireside* (produced 1803).   1803.
*Love Laughs at Locksmiths,* music by Michael Kelly, from a play by J. N. Bouilly (produced 1803).   1803.
*The Gay Deceivers; or, More Laugh Than Love,* music by Michael Kelly, from a play by Theodore Hell (produced 1804).   1808.
*The Children in the Wood* (produced 1805?).   1805.
*Who Wants a Guinea?* (produced 1805).   1805.
*We Fly by Night; or, Long Stories* (produced 1806).   1808.
*The Forty Thieves,* with Sheridan, music by Michael Kelly (produced 1806).   1808; as *Ali Baba,* 1814.
*The Africans; or, War, Love, and Duty,* music by Michael Kelly (produced 1808).   1808.
*X.Y.Z.* (produced 1810).   1820.
*The Quadrupeds of Quedlinburgh; or, The Rovers of Weimar* (produced 1811).
*Doctor Hocus Pocus; or, Harlequin Washed White* (produced 1814).
*The Actor of All Work; or, First and Second Floor* (produced 1817).
*The Law of Java,* music by Henry Bishop (produced 1822).   1822.
*Stella and Leatherlungs; or, A Star and a Stroller* (produced 1823).
*Dramatic Works.*   4 vols., 1827.

## Verse

*My Nightgown and Slippers; or, Tales in Verse.*   1797; revised edition, as *Broad Grins,* 1802.
*Poetical Vagaries.*   1812.
*Vagaries Vindicated; or, Hypocrite Hypercritics.*   1813.

*Eccentricities for Edinburgh.*    1816.

Other

*Random Records* (autobiography).    2 vols., 1830.

Editor, *Posthumous Letters Addressed to Francis Colman and George Colman the Elder.*    1820.

Reading List: *Colman the Younger* by Jeremy F. Bagster-Collins, 1946; "The Early Career of Colman" by Peter Thomson, in *Essays on Nineteenth-Century British Theatre* edited by Kenneth Richards and Thomson, 1971.

\*    \*    \*

The younger George Colman was a shrewd judge of the theatrical public's taste. As such, he earned for himself a reputation as a superior writer without ever achieving anything more than popularity. His dramatic work was of four main kinds. Firstly, he was the originator of a new kind of play (his contemporary, James Boaden, writes of "a sort of Colman drama of three acts"), in which Elizabethan blank verse and a serious theme are lightened by frequent songs and imported comic characters. *The Battle of Hexham, The Surrender of Calais, The Mountaineers,* and *The Iron Chest* are all in this style, and Colman was still ready to exploit it in 1822, when he wrote *The Law of Java.* They are plays that eased the important passage of traditional tragedy into nineteenth-century melodrama. Secondly, he wrote comedies that were generally saved by his sense of humour from conceding too much to the contemporary vogue for sentimentality. *Inkle and Yarico,* his first striking success and still an interesting piece to stage, is a comedy with songs, *Ways and Means* an imitative comedy of manners, and *The Heir at Law* shows some ingenuity in the creation of Pangloss and an ability to handle the full five-act form. *The Poor Gentleman* is too much in the mawkish shadow of Cumberland's *The West Indian,* but Colman's finest comedy, *John Bull,* merits more attention than it has received. It is robust and not at all mealy-mouthed. Thirdly, there are the ephemeral theatre-pieces, *Doctor Hocus Pocus,* a pantomime, *Blue Beard,* a spectacular, *Love Laughs at Locksmiths,* a farce, and many others. Finally, there are pieces that grew out of his work as a theatre-manager. *Poor Old Haymarket* was a prelude to the new season at the small summer theatre which he had inherited from his ailing father. It reveals a fondness for the Haymarket, and a felt sense of the difference between it and the vast patent houses. *New Hay at the Old Market* exhibits Colman's familiarity with the contemporary theatre, and furnishes us with a lot of information about it.

His autobiographical *Random Records* is honest to its title. It tells regrettably little about his final years as Examiner of Plays. He was much abused for his strictness, not least because his own light verse has prurient edges; but abuse is an inevitable concomitant of the office. Colman's Examinership was unimpressive but not malicious. The submerged tradition that he was the author of *Don Leon,* a witty and obscene poem in heroic couplets proposing an explanation of the collapse of Lord Byron's marriage, may owe its currency to a contemporary delight in taxing with immorality the official guardian of theatrical morals.

—Peter Thomson

**CONGREVE, William.** English. Born in Bardsey, Yorkshire, baptized 10 February 1670; moved with his family to Ireland, 1674. Educated at school in Kilkenny, 1681–85; Trinity College, Dublin; Middle Temple, London, 1691. Involved with Henrietta, Duchess of Marlborough, who bore him a daughter. Manager, Lincoln's Inn Theatre, London, 1697–1705; wrote little for the stage after failure of *The Way of the World*, 1700; associated with Vanbrugh in managing the Queen's Theatre, London, 1705; retired from the theatre, 1706, and thereafter, at the intercession of friends, held various minor government posts, including Commissioner of Wine Licenses, Undersearcher of Customs, and Secretary for Jamaica. *Died 19 January 1729.*

PUBLICATIONS

Collections

> *Complete Works*, edited by Montague Summers.   4 vols., 1923.
> *Works*, edited by F. W. Bateson.   1930.
> *Letters and Documents*, edited by John C. Hodges.   1964.
> *Complete Plays*, edited by Herbert J. Davis.   2 vols., 1967.
> *The Comedies*, edited by Anthony G. Henderson.   1977.

Plays

> *The Old Bachelor* (produced 1693).   1693.
> *The Double-Dealer* (produced 1693).   1694.
> *Love for Love* (produced 1695).   1695.
> *The Mourning Bride* (produced 1697).   1697.
> *The Way of the World* (produced 1700).   1700.
> *The Judgement of Paris* (produced 1701).   1701.
> *Semele*, in *Works*.   1710.
> *Squire Trelooby*, with Vanbrugh and William Walsh, from a play by Molière (produced 1704).   Revised version by James Ralph published as *The Cornish Squire*, 1734.

Fiction

> *Incognita; or, Love and Duty Reconciled.*   1692; edited by A. Norman Jeffares, with *The Way of the World*, 1966.
> *An Impossible Thing: A Tale.*   1720.

Other

> *Amendments of Mr. Collier's False and Imperfect Citations.*   1698.
> *Works.*   3 vols., 1710.
> *A Letter to the Viscount Cobham.*   1729.
> *Last Will and Testament.*   1729.

> Editor, *The Dramatic Works of Dryden.*   6 vols., 1717.

Reading List: *Congreve* by D. Crane Taylor, 1931; *Congreve the Man: A Biography* by John

C. Hodges, 1941; *A Congreve Gallery* by Kathleen M. Lynch, 1951; *Congreve* by Bonamy Dobrée, 1963; *The Cultivated Stance: The Designs of Congreve's Plays* by W. Van Voris, 1966; *Congreve* by Maximillian E. Novak, 1971 (includes bibliography); *Congreve: A Collection of Critical Studies,* edited by Brian Morris, 1972.

\*      \*      \*

William Congreve is now largely read for his plays; his poems, some of which had made his name in London by 1692, are polished and epigrammatic; he wrote translations, short lyrics, and occasional poems as well as ballads, his neat songs being perhaps his best contribution. But his first literary work of note is *Incognita,* a novel largely influenced by stage techniques. Congreve wrote it, he tells us in his *Preface,* in a fortnight; he decided to imitate dramatic writing in the plot. This is a double one with two pairs of lovers. Mistaken identities, the lovers unaware their elders have already arranged the marriages as they themselves would wish them, family feuds ultimately settled by the marriages – all of it echoes polite society and permits romantic feeling. It is finely controlled, and the comic situations bring out the sophistication with which Congreve wrote this elegant, flowing story. He told the story with obvious enjoyment and embellished it with somewhat cynical comments.

His first play was *The Old Batchelor,* a light comedy full of witty conversation, yet with undertones of reality in the character of Heartwell, the surly old bachelor who prides himself on speaking truth. He is different from the stock characters of Restoration comedy, the rakes and fops; and, of course, he is entrapped and then exposed. The situation is comic, the flippancy of Bellmour and Vainlove matched by the mockery of Belinda. And the whole play moves quickly, with a liveliness that probably owed much to Congreve's careful study of Plautus, Terence and Juvenal, as well as of Ben Jonson and the Restoration playwrights.

*The Double-Dealer* followed, a sombre play indeed, which verges upon the tragic, although it has its lively songs, its coxcombs and coquettes and its wit. Maskwell is Iago-like in his machinations and Lady Touchwood's fate, after her infamy is exposed, is hardly the stuff of comedy, however much Congreve thought comedy should expose the follies of vicious people. By making them ashamed of these faults, he remarked, it should instruct them, while delighting good people "who are at once both warn'd and diverted at the expense of the Vicious." The comedy was too black for its time, however much the reader can admire the classical skill Congreve showed in its construction, its unity of time – a few hours in one evening – and place – for the action takes place in the long gallery of Lord Touchwood's house (except for two episodes in a room opening off it). The absurdity of Mr. Brisk and Lord Froth, pert and solemn coxcombs respectively, Lady Froth, the coquette who pretends to poetry, wit, and learning, and Sir Paul Plyant, an uxorious old fool, all relieve the play's starkness, and indeed we realise Cynthia and Mellefont are convincingly in love, however she may doubt the merits of marriage. The comedy centres upon Maskwell's continuous capacity for intrigue, and the passion displayed not only by the Touchwoods but by Mellefont suggests that Congreve's concept of comedy was dominated in writing this play by satiric ambitions.

His next play, *Love for Love,* rightly brought him back to public favour. This is his best acting play; it has a clear plot, abundant absurdity, humorous characterisation, and satire in plenty. Here are the stock ingredients of the comedy of manners: youth and age in conflict, contrasts between city and country ways, questions of debts and inheritances, conversations between master and servant, intrigues and marriages, deceits and witty conversations. Foresight, with his passion for astrology, his hypochondria, and his credulity, is Jonsonian; Sir Sampson Legend, authoritarian father and self-deluding lover, matches him in comic characterisation, and is akin to one of Molière's creations.

Miss Prue, the wilful ingenue, is matched by the bluff young sailor Ben, another Jonsonian character whose "humour" is marked out by his nautical language. Scandal's affair with Mrs. Foresight follows the conventional pattern of comedy which recognises the relationship of rakes and cynical married women who enjoy intrigue; Mrs. Frail, wanting to marry Valentine for his money, is tricked into marriage with Tattle whom she despises, and Valentine marries Angelica. But he has to live down his past; she is enigmatic in her response to him until he renounces his inheritance and so proves he is not primarily interested in her wealth. The "humour, plot and satire" claimed in the Prologue are all there, but this relationship between Valentine and Angelica moves a little from Restoration conventions; a touch of idealism suddenly penetrates the cynicism of Restoration comic conventions. Wit and gallantry, Angelica argues at the end of the play, are not enough. And the idealism is, perhaps, founded upon disillusion, and upon a certain fastidiousness.

In *The Mourning Bride* Congreve tried his hand at the heroic play, that strange genre which flourished in Charles the Second's age and is somewhat baffling to us. Here we have the classical use of rhetoric and music, exalted verse, and a lively plot. Congreve exhibits his dramatic sense in welding together two themes – the love of Alphonso and Almeira, and the passion of Zara, her murder of Selim, and her suicide – against a broad background of a popular resistance movement against a tyrant. For the play is violently dramatic and arresting, its language exalted yet affective.

Congreve, who had written "An Essay Concerning Humour in Comedy" in 1695 which, as well as distinguishing between wit and humour, offers us an excellent defence of English eccentricity, was now forced into a situation where he had, in effect, to defend humour on the stage. Jeremy Collier's attack on the immorality and profanity of the English stage prompted Congreve's *Amendments of Mr. Collier's False and Imperfect Citations.* It is an example of how not to reply in anger; but it shows us something more of Congreve's attitudes to comedy: that the satirical portrayal of well bred people was justifiable if their manners were ridiculous, that the author's own ideas must not be thought the same as those of the foolish people he exposed on the stage, that passages from those plays should not be taken out of context.

There followed Congreve's most brilliant comedy, *The Way of the World*, virtually his last work for the stage. (He subsequently wrote a masque, *The Judgement of Paris*, and an "Ode for St. Cecilia's Day.") This is a complex play, revolving around marriage and money, in which information is slowly revealed, and things turn out not to be what they seem. Lady Wishfort, gullible and gulled, is finally forced to allow Mirabell and Millamant to marry, Fainall is exposed, Mrs. Marwood and Mrs. Fainall suffer. The minor characters, Sir Wilfull Witwoud the buffoon, Petulant and Witwoud the fops, the servants Foible, Mincing, and Waitwell, are all brilliantly drawn, differentiated, from their first appearance on stage, by their language and attitudes. And Mirabell and Millamant mark a new refinement; they foreshadow a new sensibility, a humane quality. And they are witty, polished, epigrammatic in speech. The whole play is sparkling and lively, it brings order out of chaos, and shows Congreve was fundamentally serious, moral, idealistic. This is an impression confirmed by the few letters of his which survive. In these his warmth of heart balances his astuteness, his taste and delicacy show why his contemporaries looked upon him with – in Steele's words – "the greatest affection and veneration."

—A. Norman Jeffares

---

**COWLEY, Hannah (née Parkhouse).** English. Born in Tiverton, Devon, in 1743. Privately educated. Married Captain Thomas Cowley c. 1768 (died, 1797); one son and one daughter. Wrote for the stage, 1776–95; as Anna Matilda engaged in poetical correspondence with Robert Merry ("Della Crusca") in *World,* 1787. *Died 11 March 1809.*

PUBLICATIONS

Collections

*Works: Dramas and Poems.*   3 vols., 1813.


Plays

*The Runaway* (produced 1776).   1776.
*Who's the Dupe?* (produced 1779).   1779.
*Albina, Countess Raimond* (produced 1779).   1779.
*The Belle's Stratagem* (produced 1780).   1781; edited by T. H. Lacy, 1867.
*The School of Eloquence* (produced 1780).
*The World as It Goes; or, A Party at Montpellier* (produced 1781); as *Second Thoughts Are Best* (produced 1781).
*Which Is the Man?* (produced 1783).   1782.
*A Bold Stroke for a Husband* (produced 1783).   1784.
*More Ways Than One* (produced 1783).   1784; as *New Ways to Catch Hearts* (produced 1783).
*A School for Greybeards; or, The Mourning Bride,* from the play *The Lucky Chance* by Behn (produced 1786).   1786.
*The Fate of Sparta; or, The Rival Kings* (produced 1788).   1788.
*A Day in Turkey; or, The Russian Slaves* (produced 1791).   1792.
*The Town Before You* (produced 1794).   1795.


Verse

*The Maid of Aragon: A Tale.*   1780.
*The Scottish Village; or, Pitcairne Greene.*   1786.
*The Poetry of Anna Matilda.*   1788.
*The Siege of Acre: An Epic Poem.*   1801; revised edition, 1810.


Bibliography: "Some Uncollected Authors 16: Cowley" by J. E. Norton, and "Cowley" by William B. Todd, in *Book Collector 7,* 1958.

*     *     *

Hannah Cowley's first play, *The Runaway,* was a country-house comedy dedicated to Garrick, who "nourished" and "embellished" it. According to *The Gentleman's Magazine* for 1809, the play was written in a fortnight; if so, Cowley wrote fluently, for it is an unusually good first effort and lasted ten seasons on the stage. Her second work, *Who's the Dupe?,* a two-act farce, became one of the most popular afterpieces of the period. Later plays, including the comic opera *A Day in Turkey,* are five-act mainpieces. The two tragedies were fairly successful – *Albina, Countess Raimond* ran for seven nights and *The Fate of Sparta* for nine – but their plots are hackneyed and their language and characters dull.

The comedies, however, are among the best of their day. *The Belle's Stratagem* was the fourth most popular mainpiece written between 1776 and 1800 and was revived as late as 1913. It mixes fast-paced comic intrigue with witty dialogue and sets off a sparkling heroine and her lover in the main plot against a more sentimental pair in the sub-plot. This pattern is often repeated in later successes like *Which Is the Man?* and *More Ways Than One.* In the latter, for example, Miss Archer recalls Letitia Hardy of *The Belle's Stratagem* and Arabella parallels Lady Touchwood; in each case, the witty heroine better reflects the tone of the play than the sober one. Occasionally the blocking action opposes a father to a daughter or ward; more often, the obstacle is the attitude of one of the principals, in which cases Cowley has the other use some "stratagem" to assure the comic resolution. These comedies and *The Town Before You*, Cowley's last play, often suggest the gaiety of earlier comedy, particularly in their dialogue and heroines. Intrigue is nevertheless prominent and sometimes central, as in *A School for Greybeards*, based on Aphra Behn's *The Lucky Chance*; it sometimes sinks into farce and sometimes produces developed characters like Lord Sparkle in *Which Is the Man?*

Cowley is a mediocre poetess. *The Maid of Aragon, The Scottish Village,* "Edwina," and *The Siege of Acre* are included in her collected works but will not bear rereading. The last-named is interesting as an epic by a woman, but Cowley's patriotism cannot excuse her couplets. As a comic dramatist she deserves to be better known. Most of her mainpieces are fresh enough in language to play successfully today. Though she draws her characters and comic situations from the large pool used by all the dramatists of the century, she chooses and combines these elements well and is usually able to vivify the stereotype. Her best characters, especially, are memorable creations.

—Frederick M. Link

---

**CROWNE, John.** English. Born, probably in Shropshire, c. 1640; emigrated with his family to Nova Scotia, where they were granted territory by Cromwell, 1656; returned to England after the Restoration when the French seized the land, 1660. Early in the reign of Charles II worked as a gentleman-usher to a lady in London; began writing in 1665; wrote for the theatre from 1671. *Died in April 1712.*

PUBLICATIONS

Collections

*Dramatic Works,* edited by James Maidment and W. H. Logan.    4 vols., 1872–74.

Plays

*Juliana; or, The Princess of Poland* (produced 1671).    1671.
*The History of Charles the Eighth of France; or, The Invasion of Naples by the French* (produced 1671).    1672.
*Andromache,* from a play by Racine (produced 1674).    1675.
*The Prologue to Calisto, with Choruses Between the Acts.*    1675
*Calisto; or, The Chaste Nymph,* music by Nicholas Staggins (produced 1675).    1675.
*The Country Wit* (produced 1676).    1675.
*The Destruction of Jerusalem by Titus Vespasian,* 2 parts (produced 1677).    1677; part 1 edited by Bonamy Dobrée, in *Five Heroic Plays,* 1960.
*The Ambitious Statesman; or, The Loyal Favourite* (produced 1679).    1679.

*The Misery of Civil War*, from a play by Shakespeare (produced 1680).    1680; as *Henry the Sixth*, part 2, 1681.
*Thyestes* (produced 1680).    1681.
*Henry the Sixth*, part 1, from the play by Shakespeare (produced 1681).    1681.
*City Politics* (produced 1683).    1683; edited by John H. Wilson, 1967.
*Sir Courtly Nice; or, It Cannot Be* (produced 1685).    1685; edited by A. Norman Jeffares, in *Restoration Comedy*, 1974.
*Darius, King of Persia* (produced 1688).    1688.
*The English Friar; or, The Town Sparks* (produced 1690).    1690.
*Regulus* (produced 1692).    1694.
*The Married Beau; or, The Curious Impertinent* (produced 1694).    1694.
*Caligula* (produced 1698).    1698.


Fiction

*Pandion and Amphigenia; or, The History of the Coy Lady of Thessalis.*    1665.


Verse

*A Poem on the Death of King Charles the II.*    1685.
*Daeneids; or, The Noble Labours of the Great Dean of Notre-Dame in Paris: An Heroic Poem*, from a poem by Boileau.    1692.
*The History of the Love Between a Parisian Lady and a Young Singing Man: An Heroic Poem.*    1692.


Other

*Notes and Observations on The Empress of Morocco by Settle*, with Dryden and Shadwell.    1674.


Bibliography: *The First Harvard Playwright: A Bibliography of Crowne* by George P. Winship, 1922.

Reading List: *Crowne: His Life and Dramatic Works* by Arthur F. White, 1922; *The Restoration Court Stage, with a Particular Account of the Production of Calisto* by Eleanore Boswell, 1932; Introduction by Charlotte B. Hughes to *Sir Courtly Nice*, 1966.

\*    \*    \*

John Crowne's strengths are his sharp characterizations and a sense of the stage as medium. A competent and successful dramatist, Crowne combined an understanding of contemporary taste with consistent ethical principles. His tragedies reflect the shifting forms and politics of his age, and his comedies the growing demand for sentimental reform. His contempt for political and religious faction, for fanaticism, and for tyranny of all sorts underlies much of his work.

Although Sir Courtly Nice is Crowne's best known character, his Sir Mannerly Shallow, Ramble, and the Molierian servant girl Isabella in *The Country Wit* and Young Ranter and Father Finical in *The English Friar* are well drawn satiric figures. Each represents a familiar London type and benefits from the tradition of humours characters while bearing wider implications. Ranter, for example, is a rake and a bully, a farcical rowdy, yet his father and society's tolerance contribute to his immorality. The characterizations benefit from lively dialogue often sprinkled with witty conceits, idiomatic phrases, and graceful sentences. Crowne writes far better than most of his peers and individualizes almost every character. Bartoline lisps, Artall delights in his wit, and Florio pretends piety in *City Politiques*. A number of characters refer to Adam, Eve, Eden, and the serpent in *The Married Beau*, and their words ("we are sons of Adam/And he ne'er got much honour by his sons") suit their morals. Although Crowne's tragedies have more conventional characters, some of them are notable. The Constable of France in *The Ambitious Statesman*, Caligula, and Atreus are merciless tyrants: Phraartes, the rational opponent of religion in *The Destruction of Jerusalem*, and Memnon, the son of the Amazon in *Darius*, are original heroes. Crowne is particularly good at pairing characters. The courageous, honorable Valerius contrasts to the posturing, mad Caligula: *The History of Charles the Eighth of France* has three heroes; Airy and Laura represent two types of irresponsibility in *The English Friar*.

Crowne's comic plots are rich in intrigue, discoveries, stage business, and satire. Laura chases Young Ranter with a sword: Surly smudges and belches upon the fastidious Sir Courtly Nice, and Florio and Artall anticipate Wycherley's Horner in feigning illness in order to gain access to other men's wives. Crowne's tragedies abound with virtuous maidens, wronged queens, noble warriors, tyrants, conspirators, and ghosts in plots familiar to any student of the heroic play. Within the conventions, however, Crowne produces some well-plotted, effective plays. He arranges Antigone's visit to her imprisoned mother immediately before the scene in which her lover finds his exiled father in a cave (*Thyestes*); he portrays Phraartes's frenzied reaction to Cleonora's death just before Titus Vespasian renounces Berenice in the interest of Titus's duty to Rome. Crowne, however, is capable of extravagant language and excessive violence. The Constable of France racks his own son on stage; Atreus serves Thyestes his son's blood and then the butchered body is displayed; Darius's ghost appears and gloats over the mangled bodies of his murderers.

In addition to his tragedies and comedies, Crowne wrote a court masque, *Calisto*, an adaptation of Racine's *Andromache*, two adaptations of Shakespearian plays, and a tragi-comedy, *Juliana*.

—Paula R. Backscheider

---

**CUMBERLAND, Richard.** English. Born in Cambridge, 19 February 1732. Educated at a school in Bury St. Edmunds, Suffolk; Westminster School, London, 1744–47; Trinity College, Cambridge, 1747–51, B.A. 1751. Married Elizabeth Ridge in 1759; 4 sons and 3 daughters. Fellow of Trinity College, 1752; Private Secretary to Lord Halifax in the 1750's, and Ulster Secretary under Halifax, 1761–62; Clerk of Reports, 1762–75, and Secretary, 1775–80, Board of Trade; retired to Tunbridge Wells, Kent. D.C.L.: University of Dublin, 1771. *Died 7 May 1811.*

PUBLICATIONS

Plays

*The Banishment of Cicero.*   1761.

*The Summer's Tale,* music by Thomas Arne (produced 1765).   1765; revised version, as *Amelia* (produced 1768), 1768; revised version, music by Charles Dibdin (produced 1771), 1771.

*The Brothers* (produced 1769).   1770.

*The West Indian* (produced 1771).   1771.

*Timon of Athens,* from the play by Shakespeare (produced 1771).   1771.

*The Fashionable Lover* (produced 1772).   1772.

*The Squire's Return* (produced 1772).

*The Note of Hand; or, The Trip to Newmarket* (produced 1774).   1774.

*The Choleric Man* (produced 1774).   1775.

*The Princess of Parma* (produced 1778).

*The Election* (produced 1778).

*Calypson: A Masque,* in *Miscellaneous Poems.*   1778; revised version, music by Thomas Butler (produced 1779), 1779.

*The Bondman,* from the play by Massinger (produced 1779).

*The Duke of Milan,* from the play by Massinger (produced 1779).

*The Widow of Delphi; or, The Descent of the Deities,* music by Thomas Butler (produced 1780).   Songs published 1780.

*The Walloons* (produced 1782).   In *Posthumous Dramatic Works,* 1813.

*The Mysterious Husband* (produced 1783).   1783.

*The Carmelite* (produced 1784).   1784.

*The Natural Son* (produced 1784).   1785; revised version (produced 1794).

*Alcanor* (as *The Arab,* produced 1786).   In *Posthumous Dramatic Works,* 1813.

*The Country Attorney* (produced 1787; as *The School for Widows,* produced 1789).

*The Imposters* (produced 1789).   1789.

*An Occasional Prelude* (produced 1792).

*The Clouds,* from the play by Aristophanes.   1792.

*The Armourer* (produced 1793).   Songs published 1793.

*The Box-Lobby Challenge* (produced 1794).   1794.

*The Jew* (produced 1794).   1794.

*The Wheel of Fortune* (produced 1795).   1795.

*First Love* (produced 1795).   1795.

*The Defendant* (produced 1795).

*The Days of Yore* (produced 1796).   1796.

*Don Pedro* (produced 1796).   In *Posthumous Dramatic Works,* 1813.

*The Last of the Family* (produced 1797).   In *Posthumous Dramatic Works,* 1813.

*The Village Fete* (produced 1797).

*False Impressions* (produced 1797).   1797.

*The Eccentric Lover* (produced 1798).   In *Posthumous Dramatic Works,* 1813.

*The Passive Husband* (as *A Word for Nature,* produced 1798).   In *Posthumous Dramatic Works,* 1813.

*Joanna of Montfaucon,* music by Thomas Busby, from a work by Kotzebue (produced 1800).   1800.

*Lover's Resolutions* (produced 1802).   In *Posthumous Dramatic Works,* 1813.

*The Sailor's Daughter* (produced 1804).   1804.

*The Death and Victory of Lord Nelson* (produced 1805).   1805.

*A Hint to Husbands* (produced 1806).   1806.

*The Jew of Mogadore,* music by Michael Kelly (produced 1808).   1808.

*The Robber* (produced 1809).

*The Widow's Only Son* (produced 1810).

*Posthumous Dramatic Works* (includes the unproduced plays *The Confession, Torrendal, Tiberius in Capreae, The False Demetrius*).   2 vols., 1813.

*The Sybil; or, The Elder Brutus* (produced 1818).   In *Posthumous Dramatic Works,* 1813.

Fiction

> *Arundel.*  1789.
> *Henry.*  1795.
> *John de Lancaster.*  1809.

Verse

> *An Elegy Written on Saint Mark's Eve.*  1754.
> *Odes.*  1776.
> *Miscellaneous Poems.*  1778.
> *Calvary; or, The Death of Christ.*  1792.
> *A Poetical Version of Certain Psalms of David.*  1801.
> *The Exodiad,* with J. B. Burges.  1801.
> *Retrospective: A Poem in Familiar Verse.*  1811.

Other

> *A Letter to the Bishop of O—d.*  1767.
> *Anecdotes of Eminent Painters in Spain During the 16th and 17th Centuries.*  2 vols., 1782.
> *A Letter to Richard, Lord Bishop of Llandaff.*  1783.
> *Character of the Late Viscount Sackville.*  1785.
> *An Accurate Catalogue of the Paintings in the King of Spain's Palace at Madrid.*  1787.
> *The Observer.*  5 vols., 1788; edited by A. Chalmers, in *British Essayists,* 1817.
> *A Few Plain Reasons Why We Should Believe in Christ.*  1801; as *The Anti Carlile,* 1826.
> *Memoirs.*  2 vols., 1806–07; edited by Henry Flanders, 1856.

> Editor, *Pharsalia,* by Lucan.  1760.
> Editor, *The London Review.*  2 vols., 1809.
> Editor, *The British Drama.*  14 vols., 1817.

Reading List: *Cumberland: His Life and Dramatic Works* by Stanley T. Williams, 1917 (includes bibliography); *Dramatic Character in the English Romantic Age* by Joseph Donohue, 1970; *Cumberland* by Richard J. Dircks, 1976.

\*       \*       \*

Richard Cumberland is better remembered as the original of Sir Fretful Plagiary in Sheridan's *The Critic* than for his own prolific output, although *The West Indian* gets a mention in most theatrical histories as an archetype of sentimental comedy. Yet Cumberland was the author of around fifty plays in most contemporary forms, including a new version of *Timon of Athens* and, in *The Jew,* an enlightened plea for its time on behalf of a persecuted people. Sensitive to criticism though Cumberland was (and as his own *Memoirs* affirms), Sheridan's satire did nothing to discourage a dramatic career which began with *The Banishment of Cicero* in 1761 and ended with *The Widow's Only Son* just a year before his death, fifty years later.

Goldsmith, in his posthumous *Retaliation,* describes him as: "A flattering painter who made it his care/To draw men as they ought to be, not as they are." And it is true that his comedies too often tended to be the "bastard tragedies" Goldsmith elsewhere dubbed them.

Yet Cumberland's first play was a true tragedy, and he also tried his hand at comic opera before attempting his first comedy, *The Brothers*, in 1769. Presumably it was the relatively favourable reception accorded this play that encouraged him to continue in this vein with *The West Indian*, whose titular hero, Belcour, blunders his good-natured but untutored way through London society, a sort of diluted, colonial version of Tom Jones.

The plot of the play is convoluted even by the standards of its time, and few of the characters do more than exemplify their required vice or virtue: but Belcour himself is strong enough to sustain a certain interest through the twists and turns of the plotting, and the Irish Major O'Flaherty, an honest soldier of fortune, serves occasionally to deflate the more sententious exchanges. If Cumberland lacked much originality, his work remains nevertheless an interesting link between sentimental comedy and melodrama, and the moral code enshrined in the one is often expressed in the exclamatory style of the other in his later work.

—Simon Trussler

---

**DENNIS, John.** English. Born in London in 1657. Educated at Harrow School, 1670–75; Caius College, Cambridge, 1675–79, B.A. 1679; awarded M.A. at Trinity Hall, Cambridge, 1683. Fellow of Trinity Hall, 1679–80, then settled in London: noted early in his career as a political pamphleteer, subsequently as a playwright, and later, most notably, as a literary critic; enjoyed patronage of the Duke of Marlborough; "royal waiter" in the Port of London, 1705–20; involved in a literary feud with Alexander Pope from 1711; lived in great poverty at the end of his life. *Died 6 January 1734.*

PUBLICATIONS

Plays

A Plot and No Plot (produced 1697).   1697.
Rinaldo and Armida (produced 1698).   1699.
Iphigenia (produced 1699).   1700.
The Comical Gallant; or, The Amours of Sir John Falstaff, from the play The Merry
    Wives of Windsor by Shakespeare (produced 1702).   1702.
Liberty Asserted (produced 1704).   1704.
Gibraltar; or, The Spanish Adventure (produced 1705).   1705.
Orpheus and Eurydice.   1707.
Appius and Virginia (produced 1709).   1709.
The Invader of His Country; or, The Fatal Resentment, from the play Coriolanus by
    Shakespeare (produced 1719).   1720.

Verse

Poems in Burlesque.   1692.

*Poems and Letters upon Several Occasions.* 1692.
*The Passion of Byblis, from Ovid.* 1692.
*Miscellanies in Verse and Prose.* 1693; as *Miscellany Poems,* 1697.
*The Court of Death: A Pindaric Poem to the Memory of Queen Mary.* 1695.
*The Nuptials of Britain's Genius and Fame: A Pindaric Poem on the Peace.* 1697.
*The Monument: A Poem to the Memory of William the Third.* 1702.
*Britannia Triumphans.* 1704.
*The Battle of Ramillia.* 1706.
*A Poem upon the Death of Queen Anne and the Accession of King George.* 1714.


Other

*The Impartial Critic; or, Some Observations upon "A Short View of Tragedy" by Rymer.* 1693.
*Remarks on a Book Entitled King Arthur.* 1696.
*Letters upon Several Occasions.* 1696.
*The Usefulness of the Stage.* 1698.
*The Seamen's Case.* 1700(?).
*The Advancement and Reformation of Modern Poetry: A Critical Discourse.* 1701.
*The Danger of Priestcraft to Religion and Government.* 1702.
*An Essay on the Navy.* 1702.
*A Proposal for Putting a Speedy End to the War.* 1703.
*The Person of Quality's Answer to Mr. Collier's Letter.* 1704.
*The Grounds of Criticism in Poetry.* 1704.
*An Essay on the Operas after the Italian Manner.* 1706.
*An Essay upon Public Spirit, Being a Satire in Prose upon the Manners and Luxury of the Times.* 1711.
*Reflections Critical and Satirical upon a Late Rhapsody Called "An Essay upon Criticism."* 1711.
*An Essay upon the Genius and Writings of Shakespeare.* 1712.
*Priestcraft Distinguished from Christianity.* 1715.
*A True Character of Mr. Pope and His Writings.* 1716.
*Reflections upon Mr. Pope's Translation of Homer, with Two Letters Concerning "Windsor Forest" and "The Temple of Fame."* 1717.
*Select Works.* 2 vols., 1718; revised edition, 1718–21.
*The Characters and Conduct of Sir John Edgar and His Three Deputy Governors.* 1720; *Third and Fourth Letter,* 1720.
*Original Letters, Familiar, Moral, and Critical.* 2 vols., 1721.
*A Defense of Sir Fopling Flutter.* 1722.
*Julius Caesar Acquitted and His Murderers Condemned.* 1722.
*Remarks upon a Play Called "The Conscious Lovers."* 1723.
*Vice and Luxury Public Mischiefs; or, Remarks on a Book Entitled "The Fable of the Bees."* 1724.
*The Stage Defended from Scripture, Reason, Experience, and the Common Sense of Mankind.* 1726.
*Miscellaneous Tracts,* vol. 1. 1727.
*Remarks upon Mr. Pope's "Rape of the Lock," in Several Letters to a Friend.* 1728.
*Remarks upon Several Passages in the Preliminaries to "The Dunciad," and in Pope's Preface to His Translation of Homer's Iliad.* 1729.
*Critical Works,* edited by Edward N. Hooker. 2 vols., 1939–43.


Translator, with others, *The Annals and History of Tacitus,* vol. 3. 1698.
Translator, *The Faith and Duties of Christians,* by Thomas Burnet. 1728.

Translator, *A Treatise Concerning the State of Departed Souls,* by Thomas Burnet.  1730.


Reading List: *Dennis: His Life and Criticism* by Harry G. Paul, 1911; *The Word "Sublime" and Its Context 1650–1760* by Theodore E. B. Wood, 1972.

\*      \*      \*


John Dennis attained greater stature as a critic than as a playwright, and it is on his criticism, chiefly, that his reputation as an arch-classicist rests. According to Pope (*Essay on Criticism*), Don Quixote (in the Georgian continuation)

> Discours'd in Terms as just, with Looks as Sage,
> As e'er cou'd *Dennis*, of the *Grecian* Stage;
> Concluding all were desp'rate Sots and Fools,
> Who durst depart from *Aristotle*'s Rules.

If the second couplet is aimed at Dennis it misses the mark. Throughout his career, Dennis (like Pope) did regard Aristotle, Horace, and other ancients as the clear, unchanging universal light of "methodiz'd" Nature in which contemporary literature should be examined; his classicism is particularly evident in the cogent attacks on *The Conscious Lovers* as a misunderstanding of traditional comedy. But – as Edward N. Hooker writes in the indispensable introduction to the *Critical Works* – Dennis was an "intelligent classicist," a man alive to the power of passion in life and art, not the dry expounder of dead rules that Pope satirized. He knew and approved Longinus on the sublime; he felt, and admitted that he felt, the sublimity of the Alps and of Shakespeare. The latter, indeed, gave him difficulties, but also brought out his critical honesty: he testified to Shakespeare's greatness as well as to his disregard of the "Rules of dramatick Composition" which Dennis espoused, and then followed his logic beyond the point where angels and prudence bad him stop. Shakespeare would have written even better had he possessed "Learning and the Poetical Art," and his plays could now be improved by remedying these defects. Dennis proceeded to "regularize" *The Merry Wives of Windsor* as *The Comical Gallant*, and *Coriolanus* ("Where Master-strokes in wild Confusion lye") as *The Invader of His Country*. Both failed.

Whenever he turned from theory to practice, in fact, Dennis struggled as if in an alien medium. He could not contrive to embody his ideas in dramatic form so as to move spectators or readers, though he tried everything, even abandoning his own critical precepts; Dennis's plays were much more hospitable to "romantic" influences such as the heroic drama than his relevant critical prose would lead one to expect. The Preface to *Rinaldo and Armida* announces a *telos* of Sophoclean terror, but the text itself is a rather entertaining hodge-podge of masque, opera, and tragi-comedy with debts to Tasso, Spenser, Dryden, and Milton ("perhaps the greatest genius" in 1700 years). It contains a song with the deathless couplet – "All around venereal Turtles/Cooing, billing, on the Myrtles" – which gives some idea of the distance between Dennis and a neoclassicist such as Addison. *Iphigenia* indulged in spectacular costumes and a mighty tempest that later occasioned Dennis's only contribution to English idiom: "They've stolen my thunder!" *Liberty Asserted*, set in Canada, features a half-breed noble savage and exhibits a fondness for rant: "These are Events surpassing all Examples;/These are th'amazing Miracles of Fate!" His few comic pieces are quite unclassical.

It is easy to see why critics and audiences did not like Dennis's plays: bombast, uncertain plotting, awkward exposition, a certain laborious lifelessness. Unfortunately the repeated failures brought out a captious streak in Dennis that allowed Pope to liken him to Appius, the irascible tyrant of one of his own tragedies.

In one overlong preface after another Dennis blamed his woes on audiences, managers, theatres, the acting, the weather, or a combination thereof, and his strictures on successful playwrights such as Steele became suspect. Dennis could not accept the verdict of theatrical audiences – whom he considered ignorant, mercantile, and debased – as final, appealing instead to the reading public, to posterity; but posterity has so far seen no reason to overturn the original decision against his plays, though it has sometimes endorsed his criticism.

—R. W. Bevis

---

**DIBDIN, Charles.**   English.   Born in Southampton, Hampshire, baptized 4 March 1745. Chorister, Winchester Cathedral, Hampshire, 1756–60. Married c. 1764, but later left his wife; associated with the actress Harriet Pitt, 1767–74: had three children by her, including the playwrights Charles Isaac Mungo Dibdin and Thomas Dibdin; later married Anne Wylde, four children. Settled in London, 1760; singer and actor from 1762, and appeared in theatres in London and the provinces; playwright and composer: wrote some 1400 songs; contract composer at Drury Lane, London, 1769–76; lived in France, 1776–78; returned to Drury Lane, 1778–81; Joint Manager of the Royal Circus, later called the Surrey, 1782–85; proprietor of the periodicals *The Devil*, 1786–87, and *The Bystander: or, Universal Weekly Expositor*, 1789–90; solo performer of "entertainments" from 1787, and had his own theatre, the Sans Souci, 1796–1805. Granted Civil List pension, 1803. *Died 25 July 1814.*

PUBLICATIONS

Plays

*The Shepherd's Artifice,* music by the author (produced 1764).   1765.
*The Mischance,* music by the author (produced 1773).
*The Ladle,* music by the author, from the poem by Prior (produced 1773).   1773.
*The Wedding Ring,* music by the author, from a play by Goldoni (produced 1773).   Songs published 1773.
*La Zingara; or, The Gipsy,* music by F. H. Barthélémon, from a play by Mme. Favart (produced 1773).
*The Deserter,* music by the author, from a play by Michel Jean Sedaine, music by P. A. Monsigny and F. A. Philidor (produced 1773).   1773.
*The Waterman; or, The First of August,* music by the author (produced 1774).   1774.
*The Cobbler; or, A Wife of Ten Thousand,* music by the author, from a play by Michel Jean Sedaine (produced 1774).   1774.
*The Quaker,* music by the author (produced 1775).   1777.
*The Comic Mirror,* music by the author (produced 1775).
*The Metamorphoses,* music by the author, from plays by Molière (produced 1775).   1776.
*The Seraglio,* with E. Thompson, music by the author (produced 1776).   1776.

*Poor Vulcan*, music by the author, from a play by P. A. Motteux (produced 1778).   1778.

*She Is Mad for a Husband*, music by the author (produced 1778).

*The Gipsies*, music by Samuel Arnold, from a play by Mme. Favart (produced 1778).   1778.

*Rose and Colin*, music by the author, from a play by Michel Jean Sedaine (produced 1778).   1778.

*The Wives Revenged*, music by the author, from a play by Michel Jean Sedaine (produced 1778).   1778.

*Annette and Lubin*, music by the author, from a play by Santerre and Mme. Favart (produced 1778).   1778.

*The Chelsea Pensioner*, music by the author (produced 1779).   1779.

*The Touchstone; or, Harlequin Traveller*, music by the author (produced 1779).   Songs published 1779.

*The Mirror; or, Harlequin Everywhere*, music by the author (produced 1779).   1779.

*The Shepherdess of the Alps*, music by the author, from an opera by J. F. Marmontel, music by Joseph Kohaut (produced 1780).   1780.

*The Islanders*, music by the author, from plays by Saint-Foix and Framéry (produced 1780).   Songs published 1780; revised version, as *The Marriage Act* (produced 1781), 1781.

*Harlequin Freemason*, with J. Messink, music by the author (produced 1780).

*Jupiter and Alcmena*, music by the author, from the play *Amphitryon* by Dryden (produced 1781).

*None So Blind as Those Who Won't See*, music by Samuel Arnold, from a play by Dorvigny (produced 1782).

*The Graces*, music by the author (produced 1782).   1782.

*The Passions*, music by the author (produced 1783).

*The Regions of Accomplishment*, music by the author (produced 1783).

*The Cestus*, music by the author (produced 1783).   1783.

*Harlequin Phantom of a Day*, music by the author (produced 1783).   1783.

*The Lancashire Witches; or, The Distress of Harlequin*, music by the author (produced 1783).

*The Talisman of Orosmanes*, music by the author (produced 1783).   1783(?).

*The Long Odds*, music by the author (produced 1783).   1783.

*The Milkmaid*, music by the author (produced 1783).

*The Saloon*, music by the author (produced 1784).

*The Statue; or, The Bower of Confidence*, music by the author (produced 1785).

*Life, Death, and Renovation of Tom Thumb*, music by the author (produced 1785).   1785(?).

*Clump and Cudden; or, The Review*, music by the author (produced 1785).   1785.

*Liberty Hall; or, A Test of Good Fellowship*, music by the author (produced 1785).   1785.

*Harvest Home*, music by the author (produced 1787).   1787.

*The Fortune Hunters; or, You May Say That*, music by the author (produced 1789).

*A Cure for a Coxcomb; or, The Beau Bedevilled*, music by the author and John Collins (produced 1792).

*A Loyal Effusion*, music by the author (produced 1794).

*A Pennyworth of Wit; or, The Wife and the Mistress*, music by John Davy (produced 1796).

*First Come, First Served*, music by the author (produced 1797).

*Hannah Hewit; or, The Female Crusoe*, music by the author, from his own novel (produced 1798).   Songs published in *Chorus of Melody*, n.d.

*The Broken Gold*, music by the author (produced 1806).

*The Round Robin* (produced 1811).

Other plays and entertainments: *The False Dervise, The Land of Simplicity, Pandora, The Refusal of Harlequin, The Razor-Grinder, England Against Italy, The Imposter, The Old Woman of Eighty;* performer in *The Whim of the Moment* and *The Oddities,* 1789, and *The Wags,* 1790 – performances continued until 1809.

Fiction

*Hannah Hewit; or, The Female Crusoe.* 1792.
*The Younger Brother.* 1793.
*Henry Hooka.* 1807.

Verse

*The Harmonic Preceptor.* 1804.
*The Lion and the Water-Wagtail.* 1809.
*The Songs,* edited by George Hogarth. 2 vols., 1842.

Other

*The Musical Tour* (autobiography). 1778.
*Royal Circus Epitomized.* 1784.
*A Letter on Music Education.* 1791.
*A Complete History of the English Stage.* 5 vols., 1800.
*Observations on a Tour Through England and Scotland.* 2 vols., 1801–02.
*The Professional Life of Dibdin, Written by Himself, with the Words of 600 Songs.* 4 vols., 1803; revised edition, 6 vols:, 1809.
*Music Epitomized.* 1808.
*The English Pythagoras; or, Every Man His Own Music Master.* 1808.

Bibliography: *A Dibdin Bibliography* by Edward R. Dibdin, 1937.

Reading List: *A Brief Memoir of Dibdin* by William Kitchiner, 1884; *English Theatre Music in the 18th Century* by Roger Fiske, 1973.

\*     \*     \*

Despite his prodigious outpouring of songs, operas, entertainments, stage histories, didactic poetry, satires, novels, and autobiography, for most of his career Charles Dibdin was a Sullivan without an appropriate Gilbert. His first and best partner and librettist was Isaac Bickerstaff with whom, from 1765 to 1772, Dibdin collaborated on about eight musical pieces for the London theatres and for Garrick's Shakespeare Jubilees (1769). He wrote all the music for the popular afterpiece, *The Padlock* (1768), and in it played the servant Mungo in blackface – the first foretaste of the nineteenth-century minstrel shows. Two of Bickerstaff's and Dibdin's musical entertainments or serenatas for Ranelagh House, *The Ephesian Matron* (1769) and *The Recruiting Serjeant* (1770), are witty, short pieces modelled after the form of *La Serva Padrona* and are still occasionally performed.

After Bickerstaff exiled himself, although Dibdin continued to write for Garrick (whom he detested) until 1776, he turned out thirty pantomimes and musical dialogues between 1772 and 1782 for Thomas King at Sadler's Wells. Dibdin's often-produced ballad opera, *The Waterman; or, The First of August,* was first played at the Little Theatre in the Haymarket. A comic opera, *The Quaker*, had one performance sloppily produced at Drury Lane in 1775, but it was not until 1777, when Dibdin was in France avoiding creditors, that the opera was successfully staged. Perpetually in debt, always quarreling with theatre managers and collaborators, constantly flirting with, but not exploring, new forms of popular entertainment, Dibdin shifted from one theatre to another. He even became a partner in a new theatre, the Royal Circus, later named the Surrey, in 1782, for which he wrote upwards of sixty works, but ended up in debtor's prison for his efforts. In 1785 he wrote the comic opera *Liberty Hall* which is remembered (if at all) for three songs: "The Highmettled Racer," "Jock Ratlin," and "The Bells of Aberdovey." Two years later he toured the country with his own one-man show to raise money for an aborted voyage to India. Typical of Dibdin's energy was his *The Whim of the Moment* (1789), one of about thirty "table entertainments" for which he was manager, author, composer, narrator, singer, and accompanist. Renamed *The Oddities* and produced at the Lyceum, it includes Dibdin's most famous song, "Tom Bowling."

At his own theatre, the Sans Souci, Dibdin introduced many of his popular, uplifting, patriotic sea songs. In all he wrote about 1,400 songs and a huge number of stage productions from puppet shows and brief musical dialogues to comic operas. Although he was awarded a £200 pension in 1803 for celebrating the bravery and loyalty of the British sailor, Dibdin's creative energies were most fully realized when he collaborated early in his career with Bickerstaff.

—Peter A. Tasch

---

**DODSLEY, Robert.** English. Born near Mansfield, Nottinghamshire, 13 February 1703. Apprenticed to a stocking weaver in Mansfield, from whom he ran away. Married; his wife died in 1754. Became a footman to the Hon. Mrs. Lowther in London, who encouraged him in his writing and secured him other patrons, including Alexander Pope; set up as a bookseller, at "Tully's Head" in Pall Mall, 1735, and subsequently published works by Johnson, Pope, and others; suggested to Johnson the scheme of an English dictionary, 1746, and was one of the publishers of the first edition, 1755; started various journals, *The Publick Register*, 1741, *The Museum*, 1746–47, *The Preceptor*, 1748, and *The World*, 1753–56; founded *the Annual Register*, initially edited by Edmund Burke, 1758; retired from bookselling and publishing, 1759. *Died 23 December 1764.*

PUBLICATIONS

Collections

*Works of the English Poets 15,* edited by A. Chalmers.    1810.

Plays

*An Entertainment for Her Majesty's Birthday.*    1732.
*An Entertainment for the Wedding of Governor Lowther.*    1732.

*The Toy-Shop* (produced 1735).    1735; with *Epistles and Poems on Several Occasions*, 1737.

*The King and the Miller of Mansfield* (produced 1737).    1737.

*Sir John Cockle at Court, Being the Sequel to The King and the Miller* (produced 1738).    1738.

*The Blind Beggar of Bethnal Green*, from the play by John Day and Henry Chettle (produced 1741).    1741.

*Rex and Pontifex*, in *Trifles*.    1745.

*The Triumph of Peace*, music by Thomas Arne (produced 1749).    1749.

*Cleone* (produced 1758).    1758.


Verse

*Servitude*.    1729; as *The Footman's Friendly Advice*, 1731.

*An Epistle from a Footman to Stephen Duck*.    1731.

*A Sketch of the Miseries of Poverty*.    1731.

*A Muse in Livery; or, The Footman's Miscellany*.    1732.

*The Modern Reasoners: An Epistle to a Friend*.    1734.

*An Epistle to Mr. Pope, Occasioned by His Essay on Man*.    1734.

*Beauty; or, The Art of Charming*.    1735.

*The Art of Preaching, in Imitation of Horace's Art of Poetry*.    1738.

*Colin's Kisses, Being Twelve New Songs*.    1742.

*Pain and Patience*.    1742.

*Public Virtue, book 1: Agriculture*.    1753.

*Melpomene; or, The Regions of Terror and Pity*.    1757.


Other

*The Chronicle of the Kings of England, Written in the Manner of the Ancient Jewish Historians*.    2 vols., 1740–41.

*Trifles*.    2 vols., 1745–77.

*The Oeconomy of Human Life, Translated from an Indian Manuscript*.    1751.

Editor, *A Select Collection of Old Plays*.    12 vols., 1744; edited by W. C. Hazlitt, 15 vols., 1874–76.

Editor, *A Collection of Poems by Several Hands*.    3 vols., 1748; revised edition, 6 vols., 1748–58; edited by I. Reed, 6 vols., 1782.

Editor, *Select Fables of Aesop and Other Fabulists*.    1761.

Editor, *Fugitive Pieces on Various Subjects*.    2 vols., 1761.

Editor, *The Works of William Shenstone*.    2 vols., 1764.


Reading List: *Dodsley, Poet, Publisher, and Playwright* by Ralph Straus, 1910 (includes bibliography).

\*        \*        \*

Footman, poet, and playwright, Robert Dodsley was the most important publisher of the eighteenth century both in terms of the men whose works he issued – Pope, Young, Akenside, Gray, Johnson, Burke, Shenstone, Sterne, among others – and in terms of the works he edited or initiated. His *Collection of Poems by Several Hands* rescued from pamphlet obscurity many of the best and most representative poems of the mid-century. *A Select*

*Collection of Old Plays* did the same for the lesser Elizabethan dramatists. His enormously successful society periodical *The World* is second in quality only to *The Spectator*; and *The Annual Register*, which he astutely contracted Burke to edit, established a tradition of excellence in assembling the best of each year's poetry and prose. A labor of love, his popular *Select Fables* included the first comprehensive, orginal study of that genre of English.

Although he is not an important poet, many of Dodsley's verses are better than his amusingly ill-considered lines "To the Honourable Lady Howe, Upon the Death of Her Husband": "But let this thought alleviate/The sorrows of your mind:/He's gone – but he is gone so late/You can't be long behind." If, in its celebration "of various Manures" and its delineation of sheep diseases, there is a turgid frivolity to the blank verse of his ambitious georgic *Agriculture*, the couplets of *The Art of Preaching*, a satire on abuses of the clergy, show facility and cleverness. The more ephemeral the subject, the surer Dodsley's touch. A few of his epigrams are excellent. "An Epistle to Stephen Duck" ingratiatingly compares Dodsley, the aspiring footman, to the thresher poet, newly called to eminence by the Queen. "Colin's Kisses," variations on a pastoral theme, are always melodious and often charming. Dodsley's one success in a more august mode – *Melpomene; or, the Regions of Terrour and Pity* – was applauded as sublime by his contemporaries, and even today the stanza and imagery of this homostrophic ode effectively present the various tragic tableaux.

Three of Dodsley's plays deserve particular mention. The plotless but good-humored *Toy-Shop* offers a satiric merchant who philosophizes over every sale. *The King and the Miller of Mansfield*, the democratically biased tale of a monarch lost in Sherwood Forest who is entertained incognito by an honest tradesman, was a theatrical triumph, establishing Dodsley as the most important sentimentalist of the 1730's. A disappointing sequel, *Sir John Cockle at Court*, reverses the premise of the original play by taking the blunt miller to London. Dodsley's greatest success and the play in which he comes closest to "the sentiment sublime, the language of the heart" which he recommends in *Melpomene* is *Cleone*, a domestic drama of traduction, murder, and madness which avoids the stilted heroics usual in mid-century tragedies. Although psychologically unconvincing, the play does achieve by flashes an authentic tragic tone worthy of Otway, to whose work Johnson compared it. Eighteenth-century audiences found the pathetic madness and death of Cleone so emotionally disturbing that Sarah Siddons had to discontinue the role.

—Harry M. Solomon

---

**DRYDEN, John.**  English.  Born in Aldwinckle All Saints, Northamptonshire, 19 August 1631. Educated at Westminster School, London (King's Scholar), 1646–50; Trinity College, Cambridge (pensioner), 1650–54, B.A. 1654. Married Lady Elizabeth Howard in 1663. Remained in Cambridge, 1654–57; settled in London, 1657, and possibly held a minor post in Cromwell's government; thereafter supported himself mainly by writing plays. Appointed Poet Laureate, 1668, and Historiographer Royal, 1669: converted to Roman Catholicism, c. 1685, and lost his royal offices at the accession of William and Mary, 1689. Member, Royal Society, 1660. *Died 1 May 1700.*

PUBLICATIONS

## Collections

*The Works,* edited by Sir Walter Scott.    18 vols., 1808; revised edition edited by George Saintsbury, 1882–92.
*Dramatic Works,* edited by Montague Summers.    6 vols., 1931–32.
*Letters,* edited by Charles E. Ward.    1942.
*Works,* edited by Edward N. Hooker and H. T. Swedenberg, Jr.    1956 –
*Poems,* edited by James Kinsley.    4 vols., 1958.
*Four Comedies, Four Tragedies* (includes *Secret Love, Sir Martin Mar-All, An Evening's Love, Marriage A-la-Mode, The Indian Emperor, Aureng-Zebe, All for Love, Don Sebastian*), edited by L. A. Beaurline and Fredson Bowers.    2 vols., 1967.
*A Selection,* edited by John Conaghan.    1978.

## Plays

*The Wild Gallant* (produced 1663).    1669; in *Works 8,* 1962.
*The Indian Queen,* with Sir Robert Howard (produced 1664).    In *Four New Plays,* by Howard, 1665.
*The Rival Ladies* (produced 1664).    1664; in *Works 8,* 1962.
*The Indian Emperor; or, The Conquest of Mexico by the Spaniards, Being the Sequel of The Indian Queen* (produced 1665).    1667; in *Works 9,* 1966.
*Secret Love; or, The Maiden Queen* (produced 1667).    1668; in *Works 9,* 1966.
*Sir Martin Mar-All; or, The Feigned Innocence,* from a translation by William Cavendish of a play by Molière (produced 1667).    1668; in *Works 9,* 1966.
*The Tempest; or, The Enchanted Island,* with William Davenant, from the play by Shakespeare (produced 1667).    1670; edited by Vivian Summers, 1974.
*An Evening's Love; or, The Mock Astrologer* (produced 1668).    1671; in *Works 10,* 1970.
*Tyrannic Love; or, The Royal Martyr* (produced 1669).    1670; in *Works 10,* 1970.
*The Conquest of Granada by the Spaniards,* 2 parts (produced 1670, 1671).    1672; in *Works 2,* 1978.
*Marriage A-la-Mode* (produced 1672).    1673; in *Works 2,* 1978.
*The Assignation; or, Love in a Nunnery* (produced 1672).    1673; in *Works 2,* 1978.
*Amboyna* (produced 1673).    1673.
*Aureng-Zebe* (produced 1675).    1676; edited by Frederick M. Link, 1971.
*The State of Innocence and Fall of Man.*    1677.
*All for Love; or, The World Well Lost,* from the play *Antony and Cleopatra* by Shakespeare (produced 1677).    1678; edited by David M. Vieth, 1974.
*The Kind Keeper; or, Mr. Limberham* (produced 1678).    1680; edited by A. Norman Jeffares, in *Restoration Comedy,* 1974.
*Oedipus,* with Nathaniel Lee (produced 1678).    1679.
*Troilus and Cressida; or, Truth Found Too Late,* from the play by Shakespeare (produced 1679).    1679.
*The Spanish Friar; or, The Double Discovery* (produced 1680).    1681.
*The Duke of Guise,* with Nathaniel Lee (produced 1682).    1683.
*Albion and Albanius,* music by Lewis Grabu (produced 1685).    1685.
*Don Sebastian, King of Portugal* (produced 1689).    1690; in *Four Tragedies,* 1967.
*Amphitryon; or, The Two Socias* (produced 1690).    1690.
*King Arthur; or, The British Worthy,* music by Henry Purcell (produced 1691).    1691.
*Cleomenes, The Spartan Hero* (produced 1692).    1692.

*Love Triumphant; or, Nature Will Prevail* (produced 1694). 1694.
*The Secular Masque*, in *The Pilgrim*, by Vanbrugh (produced 1700). 1700.
*Comedies, Tragedies, and Operas.* 2 vols., 1701.


Verse

*Heroic Stanzas to the Memory of Oliver, Late Lord Protector*, in *Three Poems upon the Death of His Late Highness Oliver, Lord Protector*, with Waller and Sprat. 1659.
*Astraea Redux: A Poem on the Happy Restoration and Return of His Sacred Majesty Charles the Second.* 1660.
*To His Sacred Majesty: A Panegyric on His Coronation.* 1661.
*To My Lord Chancellor, Presented on New Year's Day.* 1662.
*Annus Mirabilis, The Year of Wonders 1666: An Historical Poem.* 1667.
*Ovid's Epistles*, with others. 1680.
*Absalom and Achitophel.* 1681; *Second Part*, with Nahum Tate, 1682; edited by James and Helen Kinsley, 1961.
*The Medal: A Satire Against Sedition.* 1682.
*Mac Flecknoe; or, A Satire upon the True-Blue-Protestant Poet T[homas] S[hadwell].* 1682.
*Religio Laici; or, A Layman's Faith.* 1682.
*Miscellany Poems.* 1684; *Sylvae; or, The Second Part*, 1685; *Examen Poeticum, Being the Third Part*, 1693; *The Annual Miscellany, Being the Fourth Part*, 1694; *Fifth Part*, 1704; *Sixth Part*, 1709.
*Threnodia Augustalis: A Funeral-Pindaric Poem Sacred to the Happy Memory of King Charles II.* 1685.
*The Hind and the Panther.* 1687.
*A Song for St. Cecilia's Day 1687.* 1687.
*Britannia Rediviva: A Poem on the Birth of the Prince.* 1688.
*Eleonora: A Panegyrical Poem Dedicated to the Memory of the Late Countess of Abingdon.* 1692.
*The Satires of Juvenal*, with others, *Together with the Satires of Persius.* 1693.
*An Ode on the Death of Henry Purcell.* 1696.
*The Works of Virgil, Containing His Pastorals, Georgics, and Aeneis.* 1697; edited by James Kinsley, 1961.
*Alexander's Feast; or, The Power of Music: An Ode in Honour of St. Cecilia's Day.* 1697.
*Fables Ancient and Modern.* 1700.
*Ovid's Art of Love*, Book 1, translated. 1709.
*Hymns Attributed to Dryden*, edited by George Rapall and George Reuben Potter. 1937.
*Prologues and Epilogues*, edited by William B. Gardner. 1951.


Other

*Of Dramatic Poesy: An Essay.* 1668; revised edition 1684; edited by George Watson, in *Of Dramatic Poesy and Other Critical Essays*, 1962.
*Notes and Observations on The Empress of Morocco*, with John Crowne and Thomas Shadwell. 1674.
*His Majesty's Declaration Defended.* 1681.
*The Vindication.* 1683.
*A Defence of An Essay of Dramatic Poesy.* 1688.
*Works.* 4 vols., 1695.

*Critical and Miscellaneous Prose Works,* edited by Edmond Malone.   4 vols., 1800.
*Essays,* edited by W. P. Ker.   2 vols., 1900.
*Literary Criticism,* edited by A. C. Kirsch.   1966.

Editor, *The Art of Poetry,* by Nicolas Boileau, translated by William Soames, revised
    edition.   1683.

Translator, *The History of the League,* by Louis Maimbourg.   1684.
Translator, *The Life of St. Francis Xavier,* by Dominique Bouhours.   1688.
Translator, with Knightly Chetwood, *Miscellaneous Essays,* by Saint-
    Evremond.   1692.
Translator, with others, *The Annals and History of Tacitus.*   3 vols., 1698.

Bibliography: *Dryden: A Bibliography of Early Editions and of Drydeniana* by Hugh
Macdonald, 1939; *Dryden: A Survey and Bibliography of Critical Studies 1895–1974* by
David J. Latt and Samuel J. Monk, 1976.

Reading List: *The Poetry of Dryden* by Mark Van Doren, 1920, revised edition, 1931;
*Dryden: Some Biographical Facts and Problems* by J. M. Osborn, 1940, revised edition, 1965;
*Dryden and the Conservative Myth* by B. N. Schilling, 1961; *Life of Dryden* by Charles E.
Ward, 1961; *Dryden's Imagery* by Arthur W. Hoffman, 1962; *Essential Articles for the Study
of Dryden* edited by H. T. Swedenberg, Jr., 1966; *Dryden's Major Plays* by Bruce King, 1966;
*Dryden's Poetry* by Earl Miner, 1967; *Contexts of Dryden's Thought* by Philip Harth, 1968;
*Dryden: The Critical Heritage* edited by James and Helen Kinsley, 1971; *Dryden* by William
Myers, 1973; *Dryden and the Development of Panegyric* by James Dale Garrison, 1975;
*Dryden, The Public Writer 1660–1685* by George McFadden, 1978.

\*       \*       \*

John Dryden's life is largely obscure until he commences as author. He was born on 19
August 1631 at Aldwinckle All Saints in Northamptonshire, and about 1646 he entered, as a
King's Scholar, Westminster School under the famous master Richard Busby. Much later he
recalled that about 1648 he had translated Persius's third satire as a Thursday night exercise
for the school. His first published poem, "Upon the Lord Hastings," appeared in 1649; on 18
May of the following year he was admitted as pensioner to Trinity College, Cambridge,
proceeding B.A. in 1654. The next years are yet more obsucre. Some color is given to the
tradition he served the Protectorate by the publication in 1659 of the *Heroique Stanza's* on
Cromwell's death.

His career may be said to begin, however, with the Restoration, and its first period to run
from 1660–1680. Early in these years he published poems on the new order, bringing
together historical, political, religious, and heroic elements. Although such a poem as *Astraea
Redux* is inferior to the poem on Cromwell, it is more ambitious. Somewhat of the new effort
succeeds in *Annus Mirabilis,* whose year of wonders (1666) included the second naval war
with Holland and the Great Fire of London. Dryden seeks too hard to connect these diverse
events, and his execution is uneven. But it has bounding energy and is his sole fully narrative
poem till far later. His talents were being recognized – in 1668 he succeeded Davenant as poet
laureate, and in 1669 Howell as historiographer royal. By the end of this period he had
completed but not published his first poetic masterpiece, *Mac Flecknoe.* If Elkanah Settle was
its first dunce hero, Thomas Shadwell finally gained the honor. The poem assesses good and
bad art, using a mock coronation skit. Father Flecknoe abdicates for his son (Shadwell). Art,
politics, and religious matters combine with paternal love to assess both the dunces and true
drama. Flecknoe is "King by Office" and "Priest by Trade." He passes to his son *Love's
Kingdom,* his own dull play, as "Sceptre." From "this righteous Lore" comes Shadwell's

soul, his opera *Psyche*. Humor and allusion combine to establish the true canons of drama and to fix Shadwell immemorially.

*Mac Flecknoe* shows that Dryden's chief interest in these decades is the stage. After a first comedy, he turned to the rhymed heroic play, rising to the high astounding terms of the two-part *Conquest of Granada*. He approached earth thereafter. *Marriage A-la-mode* consists of a mingling of serious and comic plots especially congenial to him, and a favorite still. In the Prologue to his heroic play *Aureng-Zebe*, he professes himself "weary" of rhyme, and in *All for Love* he wrote a blank verse tragedy on Antony and Cleopatra, thought by many his finest play. His collaboration with Nathaniel Lee for *Oedipus* altered his smooth earlier blank verse style to a harsher, more various medium that appears again in his adaptation of *Troilus and Cressida*. After his enormously popular *Spanish Fryar* (1680), he wrote no plays single-handedly till 1689.

The next period, 1680–1685, is dominated by engagement with the tumultuous times. In the state of near revolution over the Popish Plot and efforts to seize power from Charles II, Dryden published *Absalom and Achitophel*, his poem most admired today. Using the biblical parallel of the plot against David (Charles), Dryden creates an epic-historic-satiric blend for the machinations of Achitophel (Earl of Shaftesbury) and his dupe Absalom (Duke of Monmouth). The Chaucer-like portraits of individuals and the personal statement on government (ll. 751–810) show Dryden in full command of a public poetry.

1682 brought Dryden further attention. *Mac Flecknoe* now first appeared in print, pirated. When Shaftesbury was released from prison by a Whig jury in November 1681, a triumphant medal was struck. Next March Dryden's one bitter poem, *The Medall*, appeared. Perhaps his anger was feigned. His usual composure is evident in *Religio Laici*, his first religious poem, which curiously begins with rich imagery and progresses to a direct, non-metaphorical style unique in his poetry. In 1684 he published one of his poems most popular today, "To the Memory of Mr. Oldham," on a young poet recently dead. In that year and the next he joined the bookseller Jacob Tonson in putting out the first two of a series of "Dryden miscellanies," collections of poetry by various hands. Charles II died, and James acceded, in 1685. Dryden celebrated these events in *Threnodia Augustalis*, his first pindaric ode after one of his finest poems, the translation of Horace, *Odes*, III, xxix.

The next period, 1685–1688, coincides with the brief rule by James II. Probably about the summer of 1685 Dryden became a Roman Catholic, and in 1687 published his second religious poem, *The Hind and the Panther*, whose 2592 lines make it his longest poem apart from translations. Its style is as complex as that of *Religio Laici* had been simple. Using sacred zoögraphy (the Hind represents Catholicism, the Panther Anglicanism, etc.), fables, myth, allusion, allegory, and the slightest of plots, Dryden sets forth a timeless version of the times, including the recent and distant past (Part I), present contentions (II), and the ecclesiastical as well as national future (III). Each part has a moving personal passage and those who have most opposed Dryden's doctrine or his fable have often called the style of this poem his finest. The poetic and personal confidence thereby implied finds expression in the ode, so praised by Dr. Johnson, on Anne Killigrew, whose small poetic abilities nonetheless may represent the artist's high vocation. Music is an equally confidently used metaphor in *A Song for Cecilia's Day*, which enacts history from Creation to Judgment.

When James fled late in 1688, and when William and Mary were invited as sovereigns by Parliament, Dryden entered into the most difficult period of his career, 1688–1694. Stripped of offices and denied full engagement with his times, he turned again to "the ungrateful stage." Two plays that now seem his greatest resulted: *Don Sebastian*, concerned with tragic fate, and *Amphitryon*, a very bleak comedy. Both deal with human identity in a hostile world. In 1691 he enjoyed a fortunate collaboration with Henry Purcell on *King Authur*, an opera. In 1694, his last play, *Love Truimphant*, featured a happy ending engineered by an unconvincing change of heart. Such doubts and sputters in these years had fullest exercise in the *Satires* of 1693 (translating Juvenal and Persius) and the Preface to *Examen Poeticum*, the third miscellany.

In the last period, 1694–1700, Dryden worked through his problems. If he could not address all his contemporaries, he could focus on individuals. In 1694 two of his finest poetic addresses appear: "To my Dear Friend Mr. Congreve" and "To Sir Godfrey Kneller." Gloom remains in both, but the gloomier "Kneller" shows chastened faith even in "these Inferiour Times," The "Congreve" bears uncanny resemblance in motif to *Mac Flecknoe*. Drama is again the topic, with comparisons again settling values. Now Dryden must abdicate and Congreve have legitimate succession, even if a usurper should sneak in for a time. The "son" merits, however, and the "father" loves.

Addresses lacked the capaciousness to adjust new strains to old hopes. Such scale was achieved in the 1697 *Virgil*. Although it and his comedies most require re-assessment, it does seem that he darkens the second half of his *Aeneis* (as if the military and the public worlds do not quite merge), and that he renders the *Georgics* even more heroically and sympathetically than Virgil to show the terms on which hope remained. His real epic was to come in cento, *Fables Ancient and Modern* (1700). It combines seventeen poems made over from Ovid, Boccaccio, Chaucer, and Homer with four solely Dryden's: those two handsome ones to the Duchess of Ormonde and to John Dryden of Chesterton toward the beginning, as also *Alexander's Feast* and "The Monument of a Fair Maiden Lady" toward the end. In redoing the *Metamorphoses* as Milton had redone the *Aeneid* in *Paradise Lost*, Dryden relates his poems by links, themes, motifs, and central subject – the human search for the good life. A serene wisdom shows that such a life can finally be gained only on Christian terms. Yet the vain and sinful race continues to endear itself to the old poet. *Fables* is once again becoming a favorite of readers as it had been for the Romantics and Dryden's own contemporaries. He died on May Day 1700 of degenerative diseases, yet calm of mind to the end.

The limitations of such periodizing are represented by its failure to allow for his constant writing in "the other harmony of prose" (Preface to *Fables*). He was by no means the modern stylist some claim. He writes in numerous styles and sometimes shows no more knowledge than Milton of modern paragraph and sentence writing. In his styles, however, he established English criticism, struggling like others before him to create the critical essay. As early as *The Rival Ladies* (1664) he found his way in use of the preface, employing a method inquisitive, devoted to current issues, and yet enough assured to deal with general principles. *Of Dramatick Poesy. An Essay* is really a dialogue, his most elaborate criticism, a semi-fiction, offering heroic debate on the proper character of drama. In the "Parallel Betwixt Poetry and Painting" (a preface to *De Arte Graphica* in 1695) we see most clearly his attempt to unite neo-Aristotelian mimesis with neo-Horatian affectivism. Once more he asserted the poet's right to heighten – to take a better or worse "likeness" and remain true, or to deal with the best "nature," unlike the scientist. In a way prescient for his career, the "Account" prefixed to *Annus Mirabilis* (1667) had placed historical poetry and panegyric (by implication satire also) under the aegis of epic. These prefaces, the *Dramatick Poesy*, and his poems as well dealt with the concept of hope for human progress, which was relatively new in England, and also introduced critical and historical principles. The element most neglected by historians of criticism was his historical understanding, which permitted him to compare and differentiate and evolve a historical relativism that would later undermine mimetic presumptions. To him we owe the concept of a historical age or period possessing its own temper or Zeitgeist, with all that such assumptions have meant to subsequent thought about literature.

Such diversity – there are over thirty plays, operas, and cantatas alone – yields to no easy summary. We can observe what joins him to, or differentiates him from, his great contemporaries – or the next century. Like Marvell, Dryden was a gifted lyric poet, although in odes rather than ruminative lyrics. Like Butler, he was a learned satirist, but where Butler degrades Dryden exalts. Like Milton, he excelled in varieties of narrative and drama, just as both also overcame crises toward the end of their lives. Dryden had what Milton lacked – wit, humor, and generosity. But his extraordinary intellectual power to liken and assimilate was incapable of Milton's higher fusion of all into a single intense reality. And where Milton, like Spenser, created an artistic language spoken by no one, Dryden like Donne and Jonson created a more natural language founded on actual speech. Born early enough to remember the outbreak of civil war (1642) and to live through four different national constitutions,

Dryden wrote of subjects that poets no longer treat directly – the most momentous events of their times. For all that, his powers took on greatness only in the second half of his life, developing to the end. He practiced every literary kind except the novel, never repeating himself except in songs for plays. He is a rare example of a writer whose finest work comes at the end of a lifetime, of a century, and of a distinct period of literature. The next equivalent of *Fables* is not heroic poetry but the novel.

—Earl Miner

---

**D'URFEY, Thomas.** English. Born in Exeter, Devon, in 1653. Settled in London; an intimate of Charles II and of James II; wrote for the stage from 1676; also composed numerous songs; Editor, *Momus Ridens; or, Comical Remarks on the Public Reports*, weekly, 1690–91. *Died 26 February 1723.*

PUBLICATIONS

Plays

> *The Siege of Memphis; or, The Ambitious Queen* (produced 1676).   1676.
> *Madame Fickle; or, The Witty False One*, from the play *A Match at Midnight* by William Rowley (produced 1676).   1677; edited by A. Norman Jeffares, in *Restoration Comedy*, 1974.
> *The Fool Turned Critic* (produced 1676).   1678.
> *A Fond Husband; or, The Plotting Sisters* (produced 1677).   1677.
> *Trick for Trick; or, The Debauched Hypocrite*, from the play *Monsieur Thomas* by Fletcher (produced 1678).   1678.
> *Squire Oldsapp; or, The Night-Adventurers* (produced 1678).   1679.
> *The Virtuous Wife; or, Good Luck at Last* (produced 1679).   1680.
> *Sir Barnaby Whigg; or, No Wit Like a Woman's* (produced 1681).   1681.
> *The Royalist* (produced 1682).   1682.
> *The Injured Princess; or, The Fatal Wager*, from the play *Cymbeline* by Shakespeare (produced 1682).   1682.
> *A Commonwealth of Women*, from the play *The Sea Voyage* by Fletcher and Massinger (produced 1685).   1686.
> *The Banditti; or, A Lady's Distress* (produced 1686).   1686.
> *A Fool's Preferment; or, The Three Dukes of Dunstable*, from the play *The Noble Gentleman* by Beaumont and Fletcher (produced 1688).   1688.
> *Love for Money; or, The Boarding School* (produced 1691).   1691.
> *Bussy D'Ambois; or, The Husband's Revenge*, from the play by Chapman (produced 1691).   1691.
> *The Marriage-Hater Matched* (produced 1692).   1692.
> *The Richmond Heiress; or, A Woman Once in the Right* (produced 1693).   1693.
> *The Comical History of Don Quixote*, 3 parts (produced 1694–95).   3 vols., 1694–96.

*Cinthia and Endimion; or, The Loves of the Deities* (produced 1696).   1697.
*The Intrigues at Versailles; or, A Jilt in All Humours* (produced 1697).   1697.
*The Campaigners; or, The Pleasant Adventures at Brussels* (produced 1698).   1698.
*The Rise and Fall of Massaniello,* 2 parts (produced 1699).   1699–1700.
*The Bath; or, The Western Lass* (produced 1701).   1701.
*The Old Mode and the New; or, Country Miss with Her Furbeloe* (produced
   1703).   1703.
*Wonders in the Sun; or, The Kingdom of the Birds* (produced 1706).   1706.
*The Modern Prophet; or, New Wit for a Husband* (produced 1709).   1709.
*New Operas, with Comical Stories and Poems* (includes *The Two Queens of Brentford, or,
   Bayes No Poetaster; The Grecian Heroine, or, The Fate of Tyranny; Ariadne, or, The
   Triumph of Bacchus*).   1721.


Fiction

*Tales Tragical and Comical.*   1704.
*Stories Moral and Comical.*   1707.


Verse

*Archery Revived; or, The Bow-Man's Excellence: An Heroic Poem,* with Robert
   Shotterel.   1676.
*The Progress of Honesty; or, A View of Court and City: A Pindaric Poem.*   1681.
*Butler's Ghost; or, Hudibras, The Fourth Part.*   1682.
*Scandalum Magnatum; or, Potapski's Case: A Satire Against Polish Oppression.*   1682.
*A New Collection of Songs and Poems.*   1683.
*Choice New Songs.*   1684.
*Several New Songs.*   1684.
*A Third Collection of New Songs.*   1685.
*An Elegy upon the Late Blessed King Charles II, and Two Panegyrics upon Their Present
   Sacred Majesties King James and Queen Mary.*   1685.
*A Complete Collection of Songs and Odes,* and *A New Collection of Songs and Poems.*   2
   vols., 1687.
*A Poem Congratulatory on the Birth of the Young Prince.*   1688.
*New Poems, Consisting of Satires, Elegies, and Odes.*   1690.
*Collin's Walk Through London and Westminster: A Poem in Burlesque.*   1690.
*A Pindaric Ode on New Year's Day.*   1691.
*A Pindaric Poem on the Royal Navy.*   1691.
*The Moralist; or, A Satire upon the Sects.*   1691.
*The Triennial Mayor; or, The New Raparees.*   1691.
*The Weasels: A Satirical Fable.*   1691.
*The Weasel Trapped.*   1691.
*A Pindaric Ode upon the Fleet.*   1692.
*Gloriana: A Funeral Pindaric Poem Sacred to the Memory of Queen Mary.*   1695.
*Albion's Blessings: A Poem Panegyrical on His Sacred Majesty King William the
   III.*   1698.
*A Choice Collection of New Songs and Ballads.*   1699.
*An Ode for the Anniversary Feast Made in Honour of St. Cecilia.*   1700.
*The Trophies; or, Augusta's Glory: A Triumphant Ode.*   1707.
*Honor and Opes; or, The British Merchant's Glory.*   1708.
*Musa et Musica; or, Honour and Music.*   1710.
*Songs,* edited by Cyrus L. Day.   1933.

Other

*The Canonical Statesman's Grand Argument Discussed.*   1693.

Editor, *Songs Complete, Pleasant, and Divertive.*   5 vols., 1719; revised edition, as *Wit and Mirth; or, Pills to Purge Melancholy,* 6 vols., 1719–20.

Reading List: *A Study of the Plays of D'Urfey* by Robert S. Forsythe, 2 vols., 1916–17; *Dates and Performances of D'Urfey's Plays* by Cyrus L. Day, 1950.

*          *          *

Thomas D'Urfey is probably best-known today for his delightful and influential collection of ballads and songs, *Pills to Purge Melancholy.* However, he was a dramatist of some consequence in his day, contributing about 30 comedies, tragedies, and operas between 1676 and 1709. He is a useful author for the literary historian, as he participated in the successive trends of contemporary drama; nevertheless, his real merit lies in the distinct individuality he achieved within his otherwise imitative productions.

With *A Fond Husband,* D'Urfey followed the influential vogue of sex-intrigue comedy established by Wycherley and Etherege, yet he peoples his landscape with grotesque "humours" characters designed for the low comedians James Nokes and Anthony Leigh. D'Urfey experienced the undoubted satisfaction of seeing Charles II in attendance at three of the first five performances of this comedy.

When Ravenscroft led the way toward farce, D'Urfey quickly turned in this direction with several plays, but in one of them, *The Virtuous Wife,* he inserted a serious presentation of female virtue, introduced by a hilarious "induction" scene in which the profligate and immoral actress Elizabeth Barry announced her refusal to play the role of a virtuous woman. Again, James Nokes scored a triumph as the elderly Lady Beardly in a farcical part.

To the phase of political satires, D'Urfey offered *Sir Barnaby Whigg* and *The Royalist.* When this vogue ended, Shadwell began experimenting with exemplary drama, to which D'Urfey contributed the two works which entitle him to a place in the history of English drama: *Love for Money* and *The Richmond Heiress.* In the former, he introduced a vulgar and realistic account of a girls' boarding school for the functional purpose of securing atmosphere by means of "local colour." The main plot-line shows a distressed heroine, who speaks in the high pathetic style, and a hero who is a "man of sense" rather than the customary town rake we associate with Restoration comedy. This hero tests the heroine and seeks dominance over her, not for sentimental reasons but for future financial security. I doubt that Stendhal would have disclaimed this play, so carefully has D'Urfey built his various ironic patterns. In *The Richmond Heiress,* D'Urfey presented several innovations. The action deals with fortune hunters, all of whom are severely ridiculed, and the play ends without a marriage of the principal characters. Also, the serious treatment of the morality of the characters and the emphasis on "The Papers" (showing legal control of the estate) suggest plays of a century later.

With the three-part *Comical History of Don Quixote,* D'Urfey followed the vogue of the bawdy which led to the famous attack by Jeremy Collier. Indecent language and incident are presented with verve and vitality. The best invention is Sancho's low-life daughter, Mary the Buxom, whose rough, coarse speeches carry vividly.

Originality appears in the two-part drama *Massaniello,* in which D'Urfey chooses prose as the language of tragedy. The harsh, realistic portrayal of a bestial mob raised to power well illustrates D'Urfey's creative skill. His plays became longer and longer, containing multiple plots, and hence can be viewed as a precursor of the coming genre of the novel.

—Arthur H. Scouten

**ETHEREGE, Sir George.**   English.   Born, probably at Maidenhead, Berkshire, c 1635. Little is known of his early life: may have studied at Cambridge University, and at the Inns of Court, London, and may have spent many years abroad: unknown when his first play was produced in 1664. Had one daughter by the actress Mrs. Barry; married Mary Arnold c. 1680. Prominent figure in Restoration London, in the circle of Sedley and the Earl of Rochester; also served the court as a diplomat: Secretary to the Ambassador to Constantinople, Sir Daniel Harvey, 1668–71; on diplomatic assignment in The Hague, 1671; Ambassador to the Imperial Court at Ratisbon (Regensburg), Bavaria, 1685–89; possibly served in Paris, 1691. Knighted c. 1685. *Died in 1691.*

PUBLICATIONS

Collections

    *Works,* edited by H. F. B. Brett-Smith.   2 vols. (of 3), 1927.
    *Poems,* edited by James Thorpe.   1963.
    *Letters,* edited by Frederick Bracher.   1974.

Plays

    *The Comical Revenge; or, Love in a Tub* (produced 1664).   1664.
    *She Would If She Could* (produced 1668).   1668; edited by Charlene M. Taylor, 1971.
    *The Man of Mode; or, Sir Fopling Flutter* (produced 1676).   1676; edited by John
       Conaghan, 1973.

Other

    *The Letterbook,* edited by Sybil M. Rosenfeld.   1928.

Reading List: *Etherege: Sein Leben, Seine Zeit, und Seine Dramen* by V. Meindl, 1901; *Etherege: A Study in Restoration Comedy* by Frances S. McCamic, 1931; *Etherege and the 17th-Century Comedy of Manners* by Dale Underwood, 1957.

*        *        *

    Although Sir George Etherege wrote only three plays, he exerted enormous influence on his successors and is usually regarded as the originator of the Restoration comedy of manners. All of his plays contain the wit and satire that characterize this kind of comedy, but it was his last and best play, *The Man of Mode,* that provided the characters, values, and language that became models for later dramatists.
    Etherege's plays depict the sophisticated, fashionable world of courtier-rakes and coquettes, and satirize the affectations and foibles of a society Etherege knew intimately. The appeal of Etheregean comedy, which is chiefly based on brilliant wit and polished dialogue, is usually intellectual, although occasional farcical elements are present, while plot complications derive from sexual and romantic intrigue.
    Each of Etherege's plays affirms a unique and complex set of values which carefully defines a hierarchy of characters and modes of behavior, and by which each character and event is measured. The action in each play centers around a battle of wits between hero and

heroine. The hero, who has not seriously considered marriage, is captured by a heroine who is the only character who fully understands the hero. The hero and heroine are contrasted with minor characters whose activities help delineate the characters of the hero and heroine. Each hero is superior to the other men in his play in that he exhibits greater knowledge of self and environment, is able to determine the proper balance between convention and nature, can manipulate his fellow-creatures to his advantage, and follows the most "reasonable" course of action circumstances allow. Each heroine is able to meet and outmaneuver the hero on his own ground, recognizes her unique limitations, comprehends the difficulty and implications of the problem she faces, and makes the hero feel that marriage is the most desirable course of action. Etherege's heroes and heroines are always evenly matched, and because they seldom face problems imposed by the external world, happiness is achieved when they overcome obstacles resulting from their own characters.

Despite these broad similarities, Etherege's plays differ significantly in structure and quality. Etherege steadily refined his art until he produced, in *The Man of Mode*, one of the most brilliant comedies in the English language.

*The Comical Revenge* contains four largely separate plots, each of which provides implicit commentary on the others. The main plot is a battle between evenly matched and resourceful lovers, Sir Frederick Frollick and Widow Rich. Comedy derives from their verbal and tactical adeptness in trying to force each other into confessions of love. The "heroic" plot is written in couplets, contains long speeches on courtly love and honor, and depicts the adventures of four lovers and a faithful friend. The two remaining "low" plots deal with the nearly successful duping of a country booby, Sir Nicholas Cully, and the imprisonment of Sir Frederick's servant, Dufoy, in a tub.

Sir Frederick and Widow Rich constitute a mean between the heroic and low plots. Love is depicted as an honorable passion, free from lust and based on purity, in the heroic plot, a conception burlesqued by Sir Frederick's continual understatement, and as a "disease" whose end-product is literally venereal disease in the Dufoy plot. Sir Frederick's concept of love is both "natural," in that it is not opposed to physical appetite and freedom, and "reasonable," in that it takes practical considerations into account. Like later Etherege heroes, Sir Frederick is able to manipulate others and to dissemble, and is generally in control of events, except those involving Widow Rich, whose self-sufficiency and resourcefulness he underestimates.

Many of the minor characters in *The Comical Revenge* are not differentiated from one another, nor is the Sir Frederick–Widow Rich plot developed as fully as the main plots in Etherege's later plays. Moreover, much of the play's humor depends on farce and burlesque, and it is not always easy to see the relationship of individual parts to one another or to the whole.

There is no heroic plot in *She Would If She Could*, but there are two sets of heroes and heroines. Characters who are able to recognize the proper relationship between social decorum and honesty are contrasted with characters entirely ruled by custom. The older, unsympathetic characters return to the country, always an undesirable place in Etheregean comedy, with the same mistaken notions they brought to town. Although minor distinctions among the four sympathetic lovers are made, the hierarchy of values is not nearly as complex as in *The Man of Mode*.

Like *She Would If She Could*, *The Man of Mode* contrasts characters who do not recognize the necessity for occasional plain-dealing with those who do, but it also contrasts those who do not understand the importance of social conventions with those who do. Characters of all shades inhabit the ground between the extremes in *The Man of Mode*. Instead of two sets of lovers, Harriet and Dorimant dominate the action of the play and regulate our response to the other characters. Dorimant is contrasted with each of the other male characters, from the completely affected Sir Fopling Flutter to such near-misses as Young Bellair, who, despite good breeding, lacks Dorimant's wit. Dorimant is acquainted with and able to profit from all fashionable modes of behavior, but is still able to maintain his identity. His only match in the play is Harriet, who is contrasted with all other women in the play, from Loveit, who sacrifices all necessary conventional restraints to emotion, to Bellinda, who, though attractive and witty, is unable to control Dorimant. Harriet's intellect, beauty, wealth, familiarity with the world, understanding of self and others, and powers of manipulation enable her to make Dorimant desire marriage. Their union represents an Etheregean ideal in which both retain individuality, freedom, and the excitement of the chase, and in which no fundamental character changes occur.

The Etheregean hero and heroine become progressively more refined in each play. Sir Frederick's drunken rowdiness is replaced by Dorimant's polished wit and naturally easy sense of propriety, much as Widow Rich's occasional coarseness gives way to Harriet's restraint and quiet aggressiveness. Sir Frederick is closer than Dorimant to the good-natured hero of sentimental comedy; in *The Man of Mode*, "good nature" can be feigned, but is not a necessary virtue.

Language is a more important source of pleasure in each successive play. In *The Comical Revenge*, language is important primarily because the sections written in couplets contrast with the prose parts; in *The Man of Mode*, Harriet and Dorimant demonstrate their superiority partially through mastery of language, and much intellectual pleasure derives from extended metaphors. In general, wit changes from frankly physical allusions to complex sexual puns and sophisticated dialogue.

The differences between *The Comical Revenge* and *The Man of Mode* illustrate Etherege's growth as a playwright. In the former, the reader is sometimes puzzled by scenes that have little relationship to preceding and following scenes, interest is divided among four plots, and our feelings about the hero and heroine are sometimes ambivalent when Etherege clearly wishes them to be positive. In the latter, plot elements are unified, our sympathies are wholly engaged by the Harriet–Dorimant relationship, and interest is fully maintained throughout by Etherege's varied and complex portrait of Restoration society.

—James S. Malek

---

**FARQUHAR, George.**   Irish.   Born in Londonderry, Northern Ireland, c. 1677. Educated at a school in Londonderry; Trinity College, Dublin (sizar), 1694–95. Married Margaret Pemell in 1703; two daughters. Corrector for the press of a Dublin bookseller, 1696; actor at the Smock Alley Theatre, Dublin, 1696–97, but gave up acting after accidentally wounding a fellow-actor; settled in London, 1697, and began writing for the stage; also an army officer: commissioned Lieutenant in the Militia, and served in Holland, 1700; Lieutenant in the Grenadiers, 1704, engaged in recruiting in Lichfield and Shrewsbury, 1705–06. *Died 29 April 1707.*

PUBLICATIONS

Collections

*Complete Works,* edited by Charles Stonehill.   2 vols., 1930.

Plays

*Love and a Bottle* (produced 1698).   1699.

*The Constant Couple; or, A Trip to the Jubilee* (produced 1699).   1700; edited by A. Norman Jeffares, in *Restoration Comedy,* 1974.

*Sir Harry Wildair, Being the Sequel of The Trip to the Jubilee* (produced 1701).   1701.

*The Inconstant; or, The Way to Win Him,* from the play *The Wild Goose Chase* by Fletcher (produced 1702).   1702.

*The Twin-Rivals* (produced 1702).   1703.

*The Stage Coach,* from a play by Jean de la Chapelle (produced 1704).   1704.

*The Recruiting Officer* (produced 1706).   1706; edited by John Ross, 1978.

*The Beaux' Strategem* (produced 1707).   1707; edited by Charles N. Fifer, 1977.

Verse

*Love and Business in a Collection of Occasionary Verse and Epistolary Prose, A Discourse Likewise upon Comedy in Reference to the English Stage.*   1702.

*Barcelona; or, The Spanish Expedition.*   1710.

Fiction

*The Adventures of Covent Garden.*   1698.

Reading List: *Young George Farquhar: The Restoration Drama at Twilight* by W. Connely, 1949; *Farquhar* by Albert J. Farmer, 1966; *Farquhar* by Eric Rothstein, 1967; *The Development of Farquhar as a Comic Dramatist* by Eugene N. James, 1972.

\*       \*       \*

Of the many comic writers who have emerged from Ireland, George Farquhar is among the very best, keeping company with such fellow-dramatists as Goldsmith and Wilde. During his short life (he died at about age thirty), he wrote eight plays (all comedies), an interesting critical essay entitled "A Discourse upon Comedy in reference to the English Stage," and some much less important miscellaneous poetry and prose. Farquhar is usually regarded as the last major dramatist writing "Restoration" comedy, but it is important to distinguish him from both his predecessors, notably Etherege and Wycherley, and his contemporaries, such as Vanbrugh and Congreve.

Farquhar's theatrical career spans the years from 1698 to 1707, which belong to a period of transition in comic drama, partly in response to increasing demands during the 1690's and early eighteenth century for more decorum and positive moral standards on the stage. The preoccupation with sexual licence, bawdry, and satire of the early Restoration playwrights, especially in the 1670's, gradually gave way to a more genteel and morally exemplary conception of comedy, culminating in eighteenth-century "sentimental" comedy. Although Farquhar's plays look back to the first masters of "wit" or "manners" comedy and are certainly not lacking in bawdy, they do exhibit features characteristic of this new tendency towards greater propriety. Most of Farquhar's heroes, for example, prove to be much less rakish in their conduct than their witty speech suggests, and they seem benevolent, good-hearted, and almost chaste in comparison to such calculating cynics and sexual athletes as Wycherley's Horner in *The Country Wife* and Etherege's Dorimant in *The Man of Mode.* Consequently critics have argued that Farquhar is more wholesome, humane, and morally nutrient as well as being emotionally softer than most Restoration dramatists. Yet this does not mean that he sacrifices comic liveliness to sentiment and sententiousness. On the contrary, there is more low comedy in Farquhar, especially in his two masterpieces, *The Recruiting Officer* and *The Beaux' Stratagem,* than in the stylistically refined though sexually squalid world of much contemporary "manners" comedy. *The Recruiting Officer* is built around an army recruiting campaign in Shrewsbury, and *The Beaux' Stratagem*, set in Lichfield, features a gang of highwaymen, prefiguring another great play of the century, Gay's *The Beggar's Opera*. Farquhar's great innovation in these, his last two plays, was to breathe new life into the conventions of Restoration comedy, which were becoming stale and outworn by the time he was writing, and he achieved this mainly by setting the actions in the provinces, not in London like most of his previous plays, and by drawing heavily on his personal experience of provincial life. The Restoration comedy of manners is virtually synonymous with London and with a small section of London Society at that, the beau monde. Characters from the provinces are almost invariably laughing-stocks because of their boorish country habits, crude speech, and ignorance of the ways of the fashionable world, and are contrasted unfavourably with modish city wits. By breaking out of the claustrophobic confines of London high society to include a much wider social spectrum, and by departing from Restoration stereotypes, Farquhar let more than a draught of fresh air into comic drama. By placing his characters in the world of small-town justices, innkeepers, tradesmen, soldiers, military recruits, highwaymen, and country wenches, Farquhar necessarily put the emphasis on humour rather than on wit, and opened up new possibilities for comedy; sadly these were not much exploited by subsequent dramatists in England, although one of the three or four great plays of the eighteenth century not by Farquhar, Goldsmith's *She Stoops to Conquer*, is certainly indebted to his example. Farquhar's real successor in this respect is the Fielding of *Joseph Andrews* and *Tom Jones*. Farquhar did, however, exert a strong influence on the development of German drama in the eighteenth century, mainly as a result of Lessing's enthusiasm for him, and even in the twentieth century he has had some impact on the German theatre; he, like his younger contemporary John Gay, was one of the British dramatists who influenced Brecht.

Farquhar's first play, *Love and a Bottle*, is an entertaining but overloaded ragbag of traditional comic devices and conventions, including mistaken identities, multiple disguises, and a complex intrigue plot. His next play, *The Constant Couple; or, A Trip to the Jubilee*, is a considerable advance, and is cleverly plotted, inventive, and full of well-drawn comic characters, yet tinged with sentimentalism. It was a great theatrical success in its first season and remained a favourite with audiences throughout the eighteenth century. Much of its popularity was due to the appealing central character, Sir Harry Wildair, who superficially resembles the rakes and libertines of Restoration comedy but differs from them in that beneath his affectation of fast-living and profligacy he is really good-natured and well-intentioned. He is unconventional, impulsive, and imprudent rather than corrupt or debauched. Encouraged by the public response to *The Constant Couple*, Farquhar wrote a sequel featuring the same principal characters, *Sir Harry Wildair*, which is even more inferior to its predecessor than most sequels. Two of his next three plays are adaptations of other plays. *The Inconstant*, based on Fletcher's *The Wild-Goose Chase* but with substantial changes, is full of broad humour and lively action. The other adaptation is the much slighter *The Stage-Coach*, a popular farcical afterpiece taken from a contemporary French play. Between these two adaptations came an original, serious, and morally explicit play upholding strict poetic justice, *The Twin-Rivals*, which differs from his previous work in its pervasive sentimentalism. In form it is a comedy, but, with its virtuous heroes and heroines, its licentious rake who is finally redeemed at a stroke, and its deformed villain, as well as its exposé of vice and evil in society, it approximates to a *drame* and falls uneasily between comedy and social-problem play.

It was after completing *The Stage-Coach* that Farquhar, now in the Army, spent some time in the provinces as a recruiting officer, visiting both Shrewsbury and Lichfield. His experiences on this mission were crucial to his artistic development, and in *The Recruiting Officer* and *The Beaux' Stratagem* he transmuted these experiences into excellent drama, at the same time revitalising the conventions of comedy. *The Recruiting Officer* contains plenty of boisterous humour, especially in the scenes satirizing corrupt recruiting methods and involving the ingenious and roguish Sergeant Kite, but at its centre is the perennial theme of comedy, love and its problems. The recruiting officer himself and the romantic hero, Captain Plume, is a descendant of Sir Harry Wildair and proves to be a man of sensibility for all his dashing military qualities, while the resourceful and practical heroine, Silvia, recalls Rosalind in *As You Like It* and Viola in *Twelfth Night*, and like them spends part of the play disguised as a young man. The triumph of romantic love over all obstacles is also a major theme of *The Beaux' Stratagem*, in which two fashionable young men-about-town, short of money and attempting to recoup their losses in the provinces, meet two country ladies and eventually fall in love with them after initially trying to trick them. Partly because the two men are mistaken for both highwaymen and Jesuits, the plot is full of comic misunderstandings and complications that give the play much of its theatrical dynamism. Both of these plays, which celebrate human vitality and variety in an almost Shakespearean way, were immediately recognised to be outstanding contributions to the genre of comedy, and time has certainly not withered their vitality and variety.

—Peter Lewis

**FIELDING, Henry.**   English.   Born in Sharpham Park, Glastonbury, Somerset, 22 April 1707; brother of Sarah Fielding. Educated at Eton College; studied literature at the University of Leyden, 1728–29; entered the Middle Temple, London, 1737; called to the Bar, 1740. Married 1) Charlotte Craddock in 1734 (died, 1742); 2) Mary Daniel in 1747. Settled in London, 1727; successful playwright, in London, 1728–37; Author/Manager, Little Theatre, Haymarket, 1737 (theatre closed as a result of Licensing Act); Editor, with James Rolph, *The Champion*, 1739–41; lawyer and novelist from 1740, also writer/editor for *The True Patriot*, 1745–46, *The Jacobite's Journal*, 1747–48, and the *Convent Garden Journal*, 1752; Principal Justice of the Peace for Middlesex and Westminster, 1748; Chairman, Westminster Quarter Sessions, 1749–53. *Died 8 October 1754.*

PUBLICATIONS

Collections

    *Complete Works,* edited by W. E. Henley.   16 vols., 1903.
    *Works* (Wesleyan Edition), edited by W. B. Coley.   1967–.

Plays

    *Love in Several Masques* (produced 1728).   1728.
    *The Temple Beau* (produced 1730).   1730.
    *The Author's Farce, and The Pleasures of the Town* (produced 1730).   1730; revised version (produced 1734), 1750; 1730 version edited by Charles B. Woods, 1966.
    *Tom Thumb* (produced 1730).   1730; revised version, as *The Tragedy of Tragedies; or, The Life and Death of Tom Thumb the Great* (produced 1731), 1731; edited by LeRoy J. Morrissey, 1973.
    *Rape upon Rape; or, The Justice Caught in His Own Trap* (produced 1730).   1730; revised version, as *The Coffee-House Politician* (produced 1730), 1730.
    *The Letter-Writers; or, A New Way to Keep a Wife at Home* (produced 1731).   1731.

*The Welsh Opera; or, The Grey Mare the Better Horse* (produced 1731).   1731; as *The Genuine Grub Street Opera*, 1731; edited by LeRoy J. Morrissey, 1973.

*The Lottery* (produced 1732).   1732.

*The Modern Husband* (produced 1732).   1732.

*The Covent Garden Tragedy* (produced 1732).   1732.

*The Old Debauchees* (produced 1732).   1732; as *The Debauchees; or, The Jesuit Caught*, 1745.

*The Mock Doctor; or, The Dumb Lady Cured*, from a play by Molière (produced 1732).   1732; edited by J. Hampden, 1931.

*The Miser*, from a play by Molière (produced 1733).   1733.

*Deborah; or, A Wife for You All* (produced 1733).

*The Intriguing Chambermaid*, from a play by J. F. Regnard (produced 1734).   1734.

*Don Quixote in England* (produced 1734).   1734.

*An Old Man Taught Wisdom; or, The Virgin Unmasked* (produced 1735).   1735.

*The Universal Gallant; or, The Different Husbands* (produced 1735).   1735.

*Pasquin: A Dramatic Satire on the Times, Being the Rehearsal of Two Plays, Viz a Comedy Called The Election and a Tragedy Called The Life and Death of Common Sense* (produced 1736).   1736; edited by O. M. Brack, Jr., and others, 1973.

*Tumble-Down Dick; or, Phaeton in the Suds* (produced 1736).   1736.

*Eurydice* (produced 1737).   In *Miscellanies*, 1743.

*The Historical Register for the Year 1736* (produced 1737).   With *Eurydice Hissed*, 1737; revised version, 1737; edited by William W. Appleton, 1967.

*Eurydice Hissed; or, A Word to the Wise* (produced 1737).   With *The Historical Register*, 1737; revised version, 1737; edited by William W. Appleton, 1967.

*Plautus, The God of Riches*, with W. Young, from a play by Aristophanes.   1742.

*Miss Lucy in Town: A Sequel to The Virgin Unmasqued*, music by Thomas Arne (produced 1742).   1742.

*The Wedding Day* (produced 1743).   In *Miscellanies*, 1743.

*Dramatic Works*.   2 vols., 1745.

*The Fathers; or, The Good-Natured Man* (produced 1778).   1778.


## Fiction

*An Apology for the Life of Mrs. Shamela Andrews*.   1741; edited by A. R. Humphreys, with *Joseph Andrews*, 1973.

*The History of the Adventures of Joseph Andrews and of His Friend Mr. Abraham Adams*.   1742; revised edition, 1742; edited by Martin C. Battestin, in *Works*, 1967.

*The Life of Mr. Jonathan Wild the Great*, in *Miscellanies*.   1743.

*The History of Tom Jones, A Foundling*.   1749; revised edition, 1749, 1750; edited by Fredson Bowers and Martin C. Battestin, in *Works*, 2 vols., 1975.

*Amelia*.   1752; revised edition, in *Works*, 1762.


## Verse

*The Masquerade*.   1728; edited by C. E. Jones, in *The Female Husband and Other Writings*, 1960.

*The Vernon-iad*.   1741.


## Other

*Of True Greatness: An Epistle to George Dodington, Esq.*   1741.

*The Champion; or, The British Mercury.*   2 vols., 1741; excerpt edited by S. J. Sackett, as *The Voyages of Mr. Job Vinegar,* 1958.
*The Opposition: A Vision.*   1742.
*A Full Vindication of the Duchess Dowager of Marlborough.*   1742.
*Some Papers Proper to Be Read Before the Royal Society.*   1743.
*Miscellanies.*   3 vols., 1743; vol. 1 edited by Henry Knight Miller, in *Works,* 1972.
*An Attempt Toward a Natural History of the Hanover Rat.*   1744.
*The Charge to the Jury.*   1745.
*The History of the Present Rebellion in Scotland.*   1745.
*A Serious Address to the People of Great Britain, in Which the Certain Consequences of the Present Rebellion Are Fully Demonstrated.*   1745.
*A Dialogue Between the Devil, The Pope, and the Pretender.*   1745.
*The Female Husband; or, The Surprising History of Mrs. Mary, Alias Mr. George Hamilton, Taken from Her Own Mouth since Her Confinement.*   1746; edited by C. E. Jones, in *The Female Husband and Other Writings,* 1960.
*A Dialogue Between a Gentleman of London, Agent for Two Court Candidates, and an Honest Alderman of the Country Party.*   1747.
*Ovid's Art of Love, Adapted to the Present Times.*   1747; as *The Lover's Assistant,* 1759.
*A Proper Answer to a Late Scurrilous Libel, Entitled An Apology for the Conduct of a Late Celebrated Second-Rate Minister.*   1747.
*A Charge Delivered to the Grand Jury.*   1749.
*A True State of the Case of Bosavern Penlez, Who Suffered on Account of the Late Riot in the Strand.*   1749.
*An Enquiry into the Causes of the Late Increase of Robbers.*   1751.
*A Plan of the Universal Register Office,* with John Fielding.   1752.
*Examples of the Interposition of Providence in the Detection and Punishment of Murder.*   1752.
*A Proposal for Making an Effectual Provision for the Poor.*   1753.
*A Clear State of the Case of Elizabeth Canning.*   1753.
*The Journal of a Voyage to Lisbon.*   1755; edited by H. E. Pagliaro, 1963.
*The Covent Garden Journal,* edited by G. E. Jensen.   1915.
*The True Patriot, and the History of Our Own Times,* edited by M. A. Locke.   1964.
*Criticism,* edited by Ioan Williams.   1970.
*The Jacobite's Journal,* edited by W. B. Coley, in *Works.*   1974.

Translator, *The Military History of Charles XII, King of Sweden,* by M. Gustavus Alderfeld.   3 vols., 1840.

Bibliography: by Martin C. Battestin, in *The English Novel* edited by A. E. Dyson, 1973.

Reading List: *The History of Fielding* by Wilbur L. Cross, 3 vols., 1918; *Fielding the Novelist: A Study in Historical Criticism* by Frederic T. Blanchard, 1926; *Fielding: His Life, Works, and Times* by F. Homes Dudden, 2 vols., 1952; *Fielding* by John Butt, 1954, revised edition, 1959; *The Moral Basis of Fielding's Art* by Martin C. Battestin, 1959; *Essays on Fielding's "Miscellanies"* by Henry Knight Miller, 1961; *Fielding's Social Pamphlets* by Marvin R. Zinker, Jr., 1966; *Fielding and the Language of Irony* by Glenn W. Hatfield, 1968; *Fielding and the Nature of the Novel* by Robert Alter, 1968; *Fielding and the Augustan Ideal under Stress* by Claude J. Rawson, 1972; *Fielding: A Critical Anthology* edited by Claude J. Rawson, 1973; *Fielding's "Tom Jones": The Novelist as Moral Philosopher* by Bernard Harrison, 1975; *Occasional Form: Fielding and the Chains of Circumstance* by J. Paul Hunter, 1975.

*    *    *

Though Henry Fielding is remembered chiefly as a novelist – as, indeed, along with Defoe and Richardson, one of the founders of the modern novel and as the author of one of the dozen or so greatest novels in English, *Tom Jones* – he began his literary career as a poet and a dramatist. A young man of twenty, without much money but with strong family connections to the Whig establishment, he came to London from the West Country in 1727 determined to make his mark as a wit and to solicit the patronage of the Court at a time when, because of the uncertain political climate following the death of George I, a talented writer might expect that his services would be appreciated by the prime minister, Sir Robert Walpole. Contrary to the usual view of Fielding as a staunch and unswerving opponent of Walpole and the Court, his earliest poems and plays reveal that when he was not actively seeking the king's and Walpole's favors he prudently adopted a neutral attitude in politics: to judge from the title of his first published work, *The Coronation: A Poem, and An Ode on the Birthday* (issued in November 1727 but now lost), he began, even in a Cibberian vein, by openly declaring his loyalty to George II; and beside several other poems soliciting Walpole's patronage in 1729–31, he dedicated to the prime minister his most ambitious, if unsuccessful, comedy, *The Modern Husband*. Indeed, as B. L. Goldgar persuasively argues in *Walpole and the Wits* (1976), of the fifteen comedies and farces which Fielding produced between 1728 – when his first play, *Love in Several Masques*, was acted at Drury Lane – and 1734 all but one were calculated shrewdly to amuse the widest possible audience without offending the Court; only in *The Welsh Opera* (1731) – a transparent political allegory satirizing not only Walpole and the leader of the Opposition, but the royal family itself – did he abandon this cautious policy, the result being, predictably, that the play was first withdrawn for revision and then suppressed.

These were the years in which Fielding established himself as London's most popular living playwright. With the exception of *The Modern Husband*, which treats rather too earnestly the disturbing theme of adultery and marital prostitution in high life, his more conventional comedies are entertaining and skillful, but by inviting comparison with the greater works of Congreve and Molière they have suffered the condescension of historians of the drama. No other critic, certainly, has endorsed Shaw's declaration that Fielding was "the greatest practising dramatist, with the single exception of Shakespeare, produced by England between the Middle Ages and the nineteenth century...." Where Fielding did shine was in the lesser modes of farce, burlesque, and satire – in *The Tragedy of Tragedies*, for example, an hilarious travesty of heroic drama, or in *The Author's Farce*, a delightful adaption of the "rehearsal play" concluding with a satiric "puppet show" performed by live actors, a work which in fact anticipates the expressionism of modern experimental drama.

Despite his reputation as the theatrical gadfly of the Court, it was only in the final three years (1734–37) of his dramatic career that Fielding moved, rather hesitantly, into the camp of the Opposition. Though he dedicated *Don Quixote in England* to Chesterfield, who had recently joined their ranks, the political satire in this play – as indeed even in *Pasquin*, which is usually said to be vehemently antiministerial – is in fact directed at the venality and incompetence of both parties. Only with *The Historical Register* and its after-piece *Eurydice Hiss'd* did he at last drop the mask of impartiality and, by ridiculing Walpole all too effectively, help to precipitate the Theatrical Licensing Act of 1737, which terminated his career as a playwright.

Forced by an Act of Parliament to abandon the stage, Fielding began preparing for the bar and, to supplement the meager income he would earn as a barrister, enlisted as a hackney author in the Opposition's campaign against Walpole. In this latter capacity, during his editorship of *The Champion* (1739–41), he almost certainly drafted his first work of fiction, *The Life of Jonathan Wild the Great*, a mock biography of an infamous real-life criminal whom he ironically praises for the very qualities of unscrupulous self-aggrandisement by which the prime minister himself had achieved "greatness." This work, however, which Walpole appears to have paid Fielding to suppress, was withheld from publication until 1743, a year after the Great Man's fall from power, when it was issued as part of the *Miscellanies*; by this time Fielding presumably had revised the novel substantially, generalizing the political satire and perhaps expanding the narrative to accommodate the more positive, contrasting element of Wild's relationship with the good-natured Heartfrees. Also included in the *Miscellanies* was *A Journey from This World to the Next*, a satirical fiction done in brisk imitation of Lucian.

It was not politics, however, but a quite remarkable literary event that provoked Fielding into finding his true voice as a novelist. Amused and not a little exasperated by the extraordinary success of Richardson's *Pamela* (1740), Fielding responded first by parodying the novel, hilariously, in *Shamela* (1741) and then by offering in *Joseph Andrews* (1742) his own alternative conception of the art of fiction. Though Fielding's improbably virtuous hero is meant to continue the ridicule of Richardson's indomitable virgin, *Joseph Andrews* is much more than merely another travesty of *Pamela*. Modelled in some respects on Cervantes' masterpiece, it yet enacts Fielding's own original theory of the "comic epic-poem in prose," whose subject is "the true ridiculous" in human nature, exposed in all its variety as Joseph and the amiable quixote Parson Abraham Adams journey homeward through the heart of England. In contrast to the brooding, claustrophobic world evoked in the letters of Richardson's beleaguered maidens, Fielding's is cheerful and expansive, presided over by a genial, omniscient narrator who seems a proper surrogate of that beneficent Providence celebrated by Pope in *An Essay on Man* (1733–34).

In *Joseph Andrews* Fielding founded, as he put it, a "new province of writing." *Tom Jones*, his masterpiece, fulfilled the promise of that ambitious, splendid beginning. Generations of readers have delighted in the comic adventures and nearly disastrous indiscretions of the lusty foundling boy who grows to maturity, discovers the identity of his parents, and marries the beautiful girl he has always loved – a story simple enough in outline, but crowded with entertaining characters, enlivened by the wit and humanity of the narrator, and complicated by the intricacies of an ingenious plot which Coleridge called one of the most perfect in all literature. Like most great books, moreover, *Tom Jones* offers us more than superficial pleasures: it is the realization of its author's profoundest philosophy of life, an artfully constructed model of a world abundant, orderly, and ultimately benign, as the Christian humanist tradition conceived it to be. Thus Fielding declares his subject to be "human nature" and his book to be nothing less than "a great creation of our own." His foundling hero stands for all of us: like the protagonists of romance, he is a kind of wayfaring Everyman who, having been expelled from "Paradise Hall," must through hard experience gain that knowledge of himself which will enable him to be united with the girl, Sophia, whose name signifies Wisdom. *Tom Jones* is, as few books have managed to be, the consummate expression of a particular form and conception of literary art.

With the publication of *Tom Jones* Fielding's life and work entered a new phase. As a reward for his services as publicist for the Pelham administration, he was appointed to the magistracy, an office which he exercised with an energy and diligence that shortened his life. His new role as a public figure, working actively to preserve the peace and to improve the wretched condition of the poor, affected his art in interesting, but most critics would say regrettable, ways. *Amelia*, his last novel, is a very different book from *Tom Jones*: Fielding's tone has become darker, more monitory, in keeping with his subject – no longer the follies of men, but their errors and cupidities and the doubtful efficacy of those institutions, the law and the church, meant to preserve the social order; his narrator less frequently appears upon the stage, and his voice, wavering between anger and a maudlin sentimentality, no longer inspires confidence. Though his ostensible focus is the domestic tribulations of the feckless Captain Booth and his long-suffering wife, Fielding's true intentions are all too patently didactic: scene after scene is calculated to expose the imperfections of the penal laws, the destructiveness of infidelity, the injustices of the patronage system, and the immoralities of an effete and pleasure-loving society. To be sure, *Amelia* is less fun to read than any of Fielding's other novels, but in the starkness and candor of its social commentary it is compelling none the less. It is in fact the first true novel of social protest and reform in England, sounding themes that would not be resumed until the next century.

—Martin C. Battestin

**FOOTE. Samuel.** English. Born in Truro, Cornwall, baptized 27 January 1720. Educated at Truro Grammar School; Worcester College, Oxford, 1737–40, left without taking a degree; entered the Temple, London, 1740. Married Mary Hickes in 1741; two sons. Jailed for debt, Fleet Prison, London, 1742–43; actor in London and Dublin from 1744; began writing for the stage in the 1740's; operated an unlicensed "lecture" theatre, London, 1762–66; lost a leg in a riding accident, 1766; granted a patent to erect a theatre: built and ran the Haymarket Theatre, London, 1766–77. *Died 21 October 1777.*

PUBLICATIONS

Collections

*Dramatic Works,* edited by John Badcock. 3 vols., 1830.

Plays

*The Auction of Pictures* (produced 1748).
*The Knights* (produced 1749; revised version, produced 1754). 1754.
*Taste* (produced 1752). 1752; revised version, as *The Diversions of the Morning* (produced 1758, and regularly thereafter), in *Dramatic Works,* 1830.
*The Englishman in Paris* (produced 1753). 1753.
*The Englishman Returned from Paris* (produced 1756). 1756.
*The Author* (produced 1757). 1757.
*The Minor* (produced 1760; revised version, produced 1760). 1760.
*Tragedy a la Mode,* from the play *Fatal Constancy* by William Whitehead (as *Modern Tragedy,* produced 1761). In *The Wandering Patentee* by Tate Wilkinson, 1795; as *Lindamira,* in *Thespian Gleanings* by Thomas Matthews, 1805.
*The Liar,* from a play by Molière (produced 1762). 1764.
*The Orators* (produced 1762). 1762.
*The Young Hypocrite,* from a French play, in *The Comic Theatre.* 1762.
*The Mayor of Garret* (produced 1763). 1764.
*The Trial of Samuel Foote for a Libel on Peter Paragraph* (produced 1763). In *The Wandering Patentee* by Tate Wilkinson, 1795.
*The Patron* (produced 1764). 1764.
*The Commissary* (produced 1765). 1765; edited by R. W. Bevis, in *Eighteenth Century Drama: Afterpieces,* 1970.
*The Tailors: A Tragedy for Warm Weather,* revised by Colman the Elder (produced 1767). 1778.
*An Occasional Prelude* (produced 1767). In *Memoirs of Foote* by William Cooke, 1805.
*The Devil upon Two Sticks* (produced 1768). 1778.
*The Lame Lover* (produced 1770). 1770.
*The Maid of Bath* (produced 1771). 1771; revised version, 1778.
*The Nabob* (produced 1772). 1778.
*Piety in Pattens* (produced 1773). Edited by Samuel N. Bogorad and Robert G. Noyes, in *Theatre Survey,* Fall 1973.
*The Bankrupt* (produced 1773). 1776.
*The Cozeners* (produced 1774). 1778.
*A Trip to Calais* (as *The Capuchin,* produced 1776). 1778.

Other entertainments: *A Writ of Inquiry; Comic Lectures; Morning Lectures.*

Other

*A Treatise on the Passions, So Far as They Regard the Stage.*    1747.
*The Roman and English Comedy Considered and Compared, with Remarks on The Suspicious Husband.*    1747.
*A Letter to the Author of The Remarks Critical and Christian on The Minor.*    1760.
*Apology for The Minor, in a Letter to Mr. Baine.*    1771.

Editor, *The Comic Theatre* (French plays).    5 vols., 1762.

Reading List: *Foote: A Biography* by Percy H. Fitzgerald, 1910; *The Dramatic Work of Foote* by Mary M. Belden, 1929 (includes bibliography); *The Life and Works of Foote* by John W. Wilkinson, 1936; *Foote, Comedian* by Simon Trefman, 1971.

\*        \*        \*

If Samuel Foote possessed the "wit of escape," as Dr. Johnson said, "in an eminent degree," he often had to employ it to escape from situations created by his wit in the first place. For most of his thirty years on the London stage Foote was something of a dramatic outlaw, "wanted" by the Lord Chamberlain's office either for evasion of the Licensing Act or slander and libel. When he emerged as a mimic in the 1740's the issue was his right to perform at all. Having no patent, Foote would invite his friends to "Tea" or "Chocolate," or (as the Examiner of Plays caught up with each name) "Diversions" or an "Auction," for which admission was charged, and then provide "free entertainment": such topical skits as a night-club comedian might devise today. Eventually this satirical pot-pourri became *Taste*. Foote was a man of many dodges, and in the end the law came over to him, so to speak: in 1766, after he had lost a leg in a riding accident, his friends procured him a summer patent at the Haymarket as a kind of disability pension. For the next few years he wrote plays around crippled heroes (*The Lame Lover, The Devil upon Two Sticks*). Long before that, however, the issue had become the angry protests of the victims of his take-offs. Virtually every one of Foote's twenty-odd plays mimicked a living individual (including George Whitefield, Thomas Sheridan, and Thomas Arne) or satirized an influential group (Methodists, nabobs, war profiteers). Usually Foote's wit extricated him from the scrape – the nabobs who came to chastise him were so charmed they stayed to dinner – or else he converted the outcry into profitable publicity; but his portrait of the Duchess of Kingston as Lady Kitty Crocodile in *A Trip to Calais* was a fatal mistake. She had the play banned, and her deputy harried Foote out of the theatre on a sodomy charge. Though acquitted, he died the following year.

Foote's extreme topicality also brought critical disapproval: only general satire of human types should be admissible and would survive, he was warned, whereas the individual eccentricities he so cruelly mimicked were by their nature ephemeral and would deservedly perish. The playwright's unfailing response was to wave the banner of Old Comedy (his favourite of many nicknames was "the English Aristophanes"). If Socrates could be spoofed on the classical Athenian stage, asked Foote, why should a modern nuisance not be pilloried likewise? He liked to think of himself as a dramatic magistrate or watchman, and of his plays as quasi-legal instruments "for the correction of individuals." Foote insisted, moreover, on calling his plays "comedies," though his contemporaries (and later critics) slighted them as "farces" and "sketches." If they are thought of as Aristophanic or *old* comedy the perfunctory and truncated plots seem less damaging, since they were merely vehicles for the main cargo of satire.

For the theatre historian Foote was an important (though not quite respectable) influence on the drama of his time. Taking up the satirical afterpiece where Fielding left off, he developed it considerably in range and style over the next three decades. Several of his long-forgotten playlets contributed stock plots and characters to Georgian comedy; Sheridan, for example, was indebted to *The Minor* and *The Author*. And perhaps the most obscure of them all was once the most influential: *Piety in Pattens*, a shrewd and amusing send-up of sentimentalism, was credited by several writers with bringing the Muse of the Woeful Countenance into disrepute just days before the première of *She Stoops to Conquer*.

To the general reader unmoved by such *arcana*, Foote can still appeal by virtue of his delight in language: not the periods of Johnson, or the wit of Sheridan, but the spoken language of the kingdom in his day. The "genius for mimicry" to which his contemporaries testified comes across now as a good ear for colloquial speech, of which Foote was a student. Although he did not hold the mirror up to nature or man, he did create a remarkably sensitive, albeit primitive, recording device, on which the voices of the men and women of Georgian England can yet be heard. The dialogue of *The Patron* and *The Commissary* remains vivid after two centuries: its tones as brash, its distortion as poignant, as an old vaudeville record.

—R. W. Bevis

---

**GARRICK, David.**  English.  Born in Hereford, 19 February 1717. Educated at Lichfield Grammar School, Staffordshire; Samuel Johnson's Academy at Edial, Staffordshire, 1736–37. Married Eva Marie Violetti in 1749. Moved to London with Samuel Johnson, 1737; wine merchant, with his brother, in London, 1738–42; appeared on the stage from 1741, and came to be regarded as the greatest actor of his age, noted for his portrayal of tragic heroes; Joint Manager, with Sheridan, Theatre Royal, Dublin, 1745–46; Joint Owner/ Manager, with James Lacy, 1747–73, and Sole Owner/Manager, 1773 until he retired, 1776, Drury Lane Theatre, London. *Died 20 January 1779.*

PUBLICATIONS

Collections

> *Poetical Works.*   2 vols., 1785.
> *Dramatic Works.*   3 vols., 1798.
> *Three Farces* (includes *The Lying Valet, A Peep Behind the Curtain, Bon Ton*), edited by Louise B. Osborn.  1925.
> *Three Plays* (includes *The Meeting of the Company, Harlequin's Invasion, Shakespeare's Garland*), edited by E. P. Stein.  1926.
> *Letters,* edited by David M. Little and George R. Kahrl.  3 vols., 1963.

Plays

> *Lethe; or, Aesop in the Shades,* from the play *An Hospital for Fools* by James Miller (produced 1740).  1745; revised version, 1757.
> *The Lying Valet,* from the play *All Without Money* by Peter Motteux (produced 1741).  1741; in *Three Farces,* 1925.
> *Miss in Her Teens; or, The Medley of Lovers,* from a play by F. C. Dancourt (produced 1747).  1747; edited by Richard Bevis, in *Eighteenth Century Drama: Afterpieces,* 1970.

*Albumazar*, from the play by Thomas Tonkis (produced 1747; revised version, produced 1773).    1773.

*Romeo and Juliet*, from the play by Shakespeare (produced 1748).    1750.

*Every Man in His Humour*, from the play by Jonson (produced 1751).    1752.

*The Chances*, from the play by Fletcher (produced 1754).    1773.

*The Fairies*, from the play *A Midsummer Night's Dream* by Shakespeare (produced 1755).    1755.

*Catharine and Petruchio*, from the play *The Taming of the Shrew* by Shakespeare (produced 1756).    1756.

*King Lear*, from the play by Shakespeare (produced 1756).    In *Bell's Shakespeare*, 1786.

*Florizel and Perdita; or, The Winter's Tale*, from the play by Shakespeare (produced 1756).    1758.

*Lilliput* (produced 1756).    1757.

*The Tempest*, music by J. C. Smith, from the play by Shakespeare (produced 1756).    1756.

*The Male Coquette; or, Seventeen Hundred Fifty Seven* (as *The Modern Fine Gentleman*, produced 1757).    1757.

*Isabella; or, The Fatal Marriage*, from the play by Thomas Southerne (produced 1757).    1757.

*The Gamesters*, from the play *The Gamester* by Shirley (produced 1757).    1758.

*Antony and Cleopatra*, with Edward Capell, from the play by Shakespeare (produced 1759).    1758.

*The Guardian*, from a play by B. C. Fagan (produced 1759).    1759.

*Harlequin's Invasion: A Christmas Gambol* (produced 1759).    In *Three Plays*, 1926.

*The Enchanter; or, Love and Magic*, music by J. C. Smith (produced 1760).    1760.

*Cymbeline*, from the play by Shakespeare (produced 1761).    1762.

*The Farmer's Return from London* (produced 1762).    1762.

*A Midsummer Night's Dream*, from the play by Sheakespeare (produced 1763).    1763.

*The Clandestine Marriage*, with Colman the Elder (produced 1766).    1766.

*Neck or Nothing*, from a play by Le Sage (produced 1766).    1766.

*The Country Girl*, from the play *The Country Wife* by Wycherley (produced 1766).    1766.

*Cymon: A Dramatic Romance*, music by Michael Arne (produced 1767).    1767.

*Linco's Travels*, music by Michael Arne (produced 1767).

*A Peep Behind the Curtain; or, The New Rehearsal* (produced 1767).    1767; in *Three Farces*, 1925.

*The Elopement* (produced 1767).

*Dramatic Works*.    3 vols., 1768.

*The Jubilee*, music by Charles Dibdin (produced 1769).    1769; revised version, as *Shakespeare's Garland; or, The Warwickshire Jubilee*, music by Dibdin and others (produced 1769), 1769; in *Three Plays*, 1926.

*King Arthur; or, The British Worthy*, music by Thomas Arne, from the play by Dryden, music by Purcell (produced 1770).    1770; as *Arthur and Emmeline*, 1784.

*The Institution of the Garter; or, Arthur's Round Table Restored*, music by Charles Dibdin, from the poem by Gilbert West (produced 1771).    1771.

*The Irish Widow* (produced 1772).    1772.

*Hamlet*, from the play by Shakespeare (produced 1772).

*A Christmas Tale*, music by Charles Dibdin, from a play by C. S. Favart(?) (produced 1773).    1774; revised version, 1776.

*The Alchemist*, from the play by Jonson (produced 1774?).    1777.

*The Meeting of the Company; or, Bayes's Art of Acting* (produced 1774).    In *Three Plays*, 1926.

*Bon Ton; or, High Life above Stairs* (produced 1775).    1775; in *Three Farces*, 1925.

*The Theatrical Candidates,* music by William Bates (produced 1775).    With *May Day,*
1775.
*May Day; or, The Little Gipsy,* music by Thomas Arne (produced 1775).    1775.


Verse

*An Ode on the Death of Mr. Pelham.*    1754.
*The Fribbleriad.*    1761.
*An Ode upon Dedicating a Building and Erecting a Statue to Shakespeare at Stratford
upon Avon.*    1769.


Other

*Mr. Garrick's Answer to Mr. Macklin's Case.*    1743.
*An Essay on Acting.*    1744.
*Reasons Why David Garrick Should Not Appear on the Stage.*    1759.
*The Diary of Garrick, Being a Record of His Memorable Trip to Paris in 1751,* edited by
R. C. Alexander.    1928.
*The Journal of Garrick Describing His Visit to France and Italy in 1763,* edited by G. W.
Stone.    1939.
*Letters of Garrick and Georgiana Countess Spencer 1759–1779,* edited by Earl Spencer
and Christopher Dobson.    1960.


Bibliography: *A Checklist of Verse by Garrick* by Mary E. Knapp, 1955; "Garrick: An
Annotated Bibliography" by Gerald M. Berkowitz, in *Restoration and Eighteenth-Century
Theatre Research 11,* 1972.

Reading List: *Memoirs of the Life of Garrick* by Thomas Davies, 1780; *The Life of Garrick* by
Arthur Murphy, 2 vols., 1801; *Garrick, Dramatist* by E. P. Stein, 1938; *Garrick* by Carola
Oman, 1958; *Garrick, Director* by Kalman A. Burnim, 1961; *Garrick and Stratford,* 1962,
and *Garrick's Jubilee,* 1964, both by Martha England; *Theatre in the Age of Garrick* by Cecil
Price, 1973; *A Splendid Occasion: The Stratford Jubilee of 1769* by Levi Fox, 1973.

*        *        *

Although David Garrick was the author of poems, prologues, epilogues, and plays, he is
remembered for his complete mastery of the British stage. His style of acting – comparatively
natural contrasted to the earlier bombast of Quin and other tragedians – broke with the old
way and began a tradition which with inevitable changes still continues. "If this young fellow
be right," Quin exclaimed, "then we have been all wrong." His success at Drury Lane proved
him right and forced his competitors at Covent Garden and the theatres in Dublin and the
provinces to follow his example of acting style and dramatic repertory. Only comic opera,
successful at Covent Garden in the early 1760's, escaped Garrick's management for a few
years until he augmented his company by inviting Covent Garden's major composer and
author to work for him. Under Garrick's and James Lacy's management, Drury Lane
prospered; when Garrick died his estate was estimated at up to £100,000.
    As a patentee of Drury Lane, and director, manager, author, and actor, Garrick tilted the
balance to a theatre dominated by the performer rather than by the author. The names
associated with the "Age of Garrick" are most likely to be those of his fellow actresses and
actors: Clive, Abington, Shuter, Woffington, Moody, King. But despite contemporary satires
which portrayed Garrick discouraging talented dramatists (as in Smollett's *Roderick*

*Random*), Garrick helped authors to rewrite their plays for a demanding but frivolous audience. As George Winchester Stone, Jr. points out (in *The London Stage*, Part 4), Garrick produced 63 new mainpieces and 107 new afterpieces during his 29-year reign. If his worst missteps were to reject John Home's *Douglas* (which succeeded at Covent Garden) and support Hugh Kelly's *False Delicacy* over Goldsmith's *Good Natur'd Man*, they are covered by the great strides Drury Lane took in stagecraft and prestige under his management.

Of the 212 different mainpieces produced by Garrick from 1747 to 1776, Stone shows that the first three of the ten most frequently performed tragedies were by Shakespeare. Of the 15 most popular comedies, three were Shakespeare's and two were by Jonson. Almost 20% of the total performances were plays by Shakespeare. Following custom, Garrick altered plays by Jonson and Shakespeare, among others, to make them vehicles for his own acting and for his repertory company, and entertaining for eighteenth-century audiences. Thus, though he did not treat *The Alchemist* or *Hamlet*, for instance, as literature, he recognized that drama must be performed if it is to be preserved. His most ambitious venture was the Shakespeare Jubilee at Stratford-on-Avon in 1769, an elaborate self-congratulatory celebration which attracted most of London's fashionable artists and their admirers. Though itself a failure, the Jubilee – at which nothing by Shakespeare was performed – can be considered one of the beginnings of Shakespearean idolatry.

Garrick's adaptations of comedies and his original farces like *The Lying Valet* and *Bon Ton; or, High Life above Stairs* amused; but *The Clandestine Marriage*, most of which was by George Colman the Elder, is an accomplished comedy unfairly overshadowed by Goldsmith's plays. Its Epilogue, a miniature comic opera by Garrick, satirizes fashionable playgoers and their infatuation with comic opera; it epitomizes Garrick's skill at light verse and bantering dialogue.

Of the over ninety roles which Garrick performed, among his most famous were Ranger (*Suspicious Husband*, Hoadly), Abel Drugger (*Alchemist*, Jonson), Hamlet and Lear, Benedick (*Much Ado*, Shakespeare), Archer and Scrub (*Beaux' Stratagem*, Farquhar), Don Felix (*The Wonder*, Centlivre), and Bayes (*The Rehearsal*, Villiers). On stage, departing from tradition, Garrick remained in character even when other performers spoke. Whatever the role, Frederick Grimm wrote in 1765, Garrick "abandons his own personality, and puts himself in the situation of him he has to represent ... he ceases to be Garrick." Of "middle stature, small rather than big," Garrick's "vivacity is extreme." Unlike many other actors, Garrick could switch from tragedy to comedy; but whether he was Richard III or Sir John Brute in Vanbrugh's *Provok'd Wife*, Garrick's "negative capability" enabled him to convince his audience that he had become that person.

Now, when actors have been knighted and performers are often associated with American politics, it might be easy to minimize Garrick's importance. But like Samuel Johnson, Garrick was an arbiter of taste. Sterne turned to him for early approval of *Tristram Shandy*, as well he should have since Garrick held shares in two London newspapers, *St. James Chronicle* (which he helped found with the elder Colman and others) and the *Public Advertiser*; his enemies accused him of being a censor-general of London's press. Artists like Reynolds and Hogarth caught his naturalness on canvas, and Goldsmith, Burke, and others of the Literary Club counted him a member. "In his time," concluded one of his early biographers, Arthur Murphy, "the theatre engrossed the minds of men to such a degree that it may now be said there existed in England a *fourth estate*, King, Lords, and Commons, and *Drury-Lane playhouse*." His funeral was magnificent; appropriately, Garrick was buried in the Poets' Corner at the foot of Shakespeare's monument. Summarizing Garrick's career, Burke wrote, "He raised the character of his profession to the rank of a liberal art."

—Peter A. Tasch

**GAY, John.**   English.   Born in Barnstaple, Devon, baptized 16 September 1685. Educated at the free grammar school in Barnstaple; apprenticed to a silk mercer in London. Secretary to the household of the Duchess of Monmouth, 1712–14; Secretary to the Earl of Clarendon on his diplomatic mission to Hanover, 1714; accompanied William Pulteney, later Earl of Bath, to Aix, 1717; lived at Lord Harcourt's estate in Oxfordshire, 1718; earned considerable income from publication of his collected poems, 1720, and made and lost a fortune in South Sea funds speculation; Commissioner for the Public Lottery, 1722–31; recovered much of his fortune from the success of the *Beggar's Opera*, 1728; lived with his patrons the Duke and Duchess of Queensberry, 1728–32. *Died 4 December 1732.*

PUBLICATIONS

Collections

*Poetical, Dramatic, and Miscellaneous Works.*   6 vols., 1795.
*Plays.*   2 vols., 1923.
*Poetical Works*, edited by G. C. Faber.   1926.
*Letters*, edited by Chester F. Burgess.   1966.
*Poetry and Prose*, edited by Vinton A. Dearing and Charles Beckwith.   2 vols., 1974.
*Selected Works*, edited by Samuel Joseloff.   1976.

Plays

*The Mohocks.*   1712.
*The Wife of Bath* (produced 1713).   1713; revised version (produced 1730), 1730.
*The What D'ye Call It* (produced 1715).   1715.
*Three Hours after Marriage*, with Pope and Arbuthnot (produced 1717).   1717; revised version, in *Supplement to the Works of Pope*, 1757; 1717 edition edited by Richard Morton and William Peterson, 1961.
*Acis and Galatea*, music by Handel (produced 1719).   1732.
*Dione*, in *Poems on Several Occasions.*   1720.
*The Captives* (produced 1724).   1724.
*The Beggar's Opera* (produced 1728).   1728; edited by Peter Lewis, 1973.
*Polly, Being the 2nd Part of The Beggar's Opera* (version revised by Colman the Elder produced 1777).   1729; in *Poetical Works*, 1926.
*Achilles* (produced 1733).   1733.
*The Distressed Wife* (produced 1734).   1743; as *The Modern Wife* (produced 1771).
*The Rehearsal at Goatham.*   1754.

Verse

*Wine.*   1708.
*Rural Sports.*   1713; revised edition, 1720; edited by O. Culbertson, 1930.
*The Fan.*   1714.
*The Shepherd's Week.*   1714.
*A Letter to a Lady.*   1714.
*Two Epistles, One to the Earl of Burlington, The Other to a Lady.*   1715(?).
*Trivia; or, The Art of Walking the Streets of London.*   1716.
*Horace, epode iv, Imitated.*   1717(?).

*The Poor Shepherd.*    1720(?).
*Poems on Several Occasions.*    2 vols., 1720.
*A Panegyrical Epistle to Mr. Thomas Snow.*    1721.
*An Epistle to Her Grace Henrietta Duchess of Marlborough.*    1722.
*A Poem Addressed to the Quidnunc's.*    1724.
*Blueskin's Ballad.*    1725.
*To a Lady on Her Passion for Old China.*    1725.
*Daphnis and Cloe.*    1725(?).
*Molly Mog.*    1726.
*Fables.*    2 vols., 1727–38; edited by Vinton A. Dearing, 1967.
*Some Unpublished Translations from Ariosto,* edited by J. D. Bruce.    1910.


Other

*The Present State of Wit.*    1711.
*An Argument Proving That the Present Mohocks and Hawkubites Are the Gog and Magog Mentioned in the Revelations.*    1712.


Bibliography: in *Poetical Works,* 1926; *Gay: An Annotated Checklist of Criticism* by Julie T. Klein, 1973.

Reading List: *Gay, Favorite of the Wits* by William H. Irving, 1940; *Gay, Social Critic* by Sven M. Armens, 1954; *Gay* by Oliver Warner, 1964; *Gay* by Patricia M. Spacks, 1965.

*          *          *

Although John Gay was one of the most talented English writers in the first third of the eighteenth century, he is overshadowed by his two close friends and fellow-members of the Scriblerus Club, Swift and Pope. Comparisons with the two literary giants of the period are therefore inevitable and usually to Gay's detriment, which is unfortunate since his gifts are significantly different from theirs. It is unfair to think of Gay as a lesser Swift or a lesser Pope. Gay certainly lacks the emotional intensity, intellectual power, and penetrating insight of Swift's great satires, and rarely equals Pope in refined verbal wit, imaginative inventiveness, and incisive irony. The all-embracing cultural survey of *Gulliver's Travels* or even the moral breadth of Pope's *Moral Essays* and *Imitations of Horace* were beyond Gay, as were the gloomy visionary quality and sustained mock-heroic elaboration of *The Dunciad.* Gay's mature work does not seem to stem from a firm ideological foundation of inter-connected philosophical ideas, political convictions and moral values in the way that Swift's and Pope's do. Nevertheless Swift and Pope are not the measure of all Augustan writers as they are sometimes thought to be, and Gay, although influenced by his two friends, usually followed his own creative impulses and did not attempt to do what they were doing. As a result he acquired a distinctive literary voice, less relentless and angry than Swift's, less acerbic and barbed than Pope's, more genial, warm-hearted and gentle than both. His satirical and burlesque works, for example, are less single-minded than theirs, so that his ridicule is often tempered with sentiment, producing a bitter-sweet amalgam that is very much Gay's own and that is particularly evident in his masterpiece, *The Beggar's Opera.* Furthermore Gay, with his less fixed intellectual commitment, was much more chameleon-like than his friends, which helps to explain the extraordinary diversity of his output.

In addition to being a versatile poet, he was a fairly prolific playwright in both verse and prose, and the only member of the Scriblerus Club to devote himself to drama. Indeed it is as the author of *The Beggar's Opera* that he is best remembered today. As a dramatist he did not restrict himself to the "regular" and neoclassically respectable genres of tragedy and comedy but attempted most of the theatrical forms of the period; and with *The Beggar's Opera* he actually invented the ballad opera, which became very popular in the eighteenth century and is the precursor of English comic opera and of the modern musical, as well as being an important influence on Brecht. Gay began his dramatic career with a short farce, *The Mohocks*, and followed this with an undistinguished comedy based on Chaucer, *The Wife of Bath*, before turning his hand to two very different satirical plays. The popular *The What D'Ye Call It* is a fine burlesque of contemporary tragedy, especially "pathetic" plays, that succeeds in transcending burlesque, while the controversial *Three Hours after Marriage*, written as a Scriblerian enterprise with Pope and Arbuthnot, is a lively and frequently farcical dramatic satire attacking a number of well-known contemporary intellectuals and artists. Not long after this he provided Handel with a libretto for his pastoral opera *Acis and Galatea* and then made two not particularly successful attempts at tragedy, *Dione*, written in couplets and in a pastoral and sentimental vein, and *The Captives*, a blank-verse tragedy in a more heroic manner that ends happily with virtue rewarded and poetic justice established. Next came by far his greatest theatrical success, *The Beggar's Opera*, a truly original work of genius and one of the very few eighteenth-century plays to hold the stage until the present day. By using a mixture of speech and song and by providing his own words for well-known tunes, Gay created a new kind of music theatre, the ballad opera, while simultaneously burlesquing Italian opera, which was enjoying a vogue in England. In addition *The Beggar's Opera*, set in the London underworld, is a most unusual love story, both romantic and anti-romantic, as well as a pungently ironic social and political satire. Amazingly enough, Gay was able to weld these diverse elements together into a unified work of art that manages to be both highly topical and universal. After the unprecedented commercial success of *The Beggar's Opera*, Gay wrote an inferior sequel, *Polly*, which was banned from the stage by the Government, offended by the scathing political ridicule of its predecessor. None of his three posthumous plays, *Achilles*, a farcical treatment of a classical legend in ballad-opera form, and the two satirical comedies, *The Distress'd Wife* and *The Rehearsal at Goatham*, adds much to his dramatic achievement.

The range and variety of his dramatic work is matched by that of his poetry, although the quality is again decidedly uneven. He wrote mock-heroic poetry, notably *The Fan*, which is indebted to *The Rape of the Lock*; an extended georgic in the manner of Virgil, *Rural Sports*; a group of pastoral poems, *The Shepherd's Week*, which burlesque Ambrose Philips's *Pastorals* yet are much more than burlesque; a long mock-georgic about London life, laced with acute social observations, guide-book advice and moral precepts, *Trivia; or, The Art of Walking the Streets of London*; a number of urbane verse *Epistles* to friends on various topics; a set of ironic Eclogues, mainly Town Eclogues about fashionable women and love; two series of *Fables* in the manner of Aesop and La Fontaine; various narrative poems, including bawdy tales inspired by Chaucer's *fabliaux*; a few meditative poems such as "A Contemplation on Night" (1714); some lyrics and ballads including the well-known "Sweet William's Farewell to Black-ey'd Susan" (1720); and translations of Ovid and Ariosto. Although much of his poetry is written in decasyllabic couplets, the standard form of the time, Gay is again more varied than many of his contemporaries since he uses the lighter and racier octosyllabic couplets for the *Fables* and some of the tales, blank verse for his early mock-heroic *Wine*, *ottava rima* for one of his Epistles, "Mr. Pope's Welcome from Greece," and a variety of stanza forms for his songs and ballads. His finest poetic achievement is the first series of *Fables*, ostensibly written to entertain a young member of the Royal Family but, as in the case of earlier fable literature, having a much wider moral, social, and political significance than the apparently innocuous subject-matter suggests. Gay's *Fables* are not of the supreme quality of La Fontaine's, but they remain the best examples of their kind in English since Henryson's admirable adaptations of Aesop into Middle Scots. *Trivia*, which has been claimed to be the finest poem about London in the language, is also a genuinely individual work revealing some of his best qualities: his observant eye for detail, his great sympathy for ordinary humanity, his down-to-earth good sense, his sturdy versification, and plain, unfussy diction. *The Shepherd's Week* is probably the most important Augustan contribution to the genre of pastoral. Much of Gay's work is now of interest only to the specialist, but in a few cases, notably the *Fables* and above all *The Beggar's Opera*, he transcends his own time and must therefore rank as a major Augustan writer.

—Peter Lewis

---

**GOLDSMITH, Oliver.**   Irish.   Born in Pallas, near Ballymahon, Longford, 10 November 1728. Educated at the village school in Lissoy, West Meath, 1734–37; Elphin School, 1738; a school in Athlone, 1739–41, and in Edgeworthstown, Longford, 1741–44; Trinity College, Dublin (sizar), 1745–49 (Smyth exhibitioner, 1747), B.A. 1749; studied medicine at the University of Edinburgh, 1752–53; travelled on the Continent, in Switzerland, Italy, and France, 1753–56, and may have obtained a medical degree. Settled in London, 1756; tried unsuccessfully to support himself as a physician in Southwark; worked as an usher in Dr. Milner's classical academy in Peckham, 1756, and as a writer for Ralph Griffiths, proprietor of the *Monthly Review*, 1757–58; Editor, *The Bee*, 1759; contributed to the *British Magazine*, 1760; Editor, *The Lady's Magazine*, 1761; also worked for the publisher Edward Newbery: worked as a proof-reader and preface writer, contributed to the *Public Ledger*, 1760, and prepared a *Compendium of Biography*, 7 volumes, 1762; after 1763 earned increasingly substantial sums from his own writing; one of the founder members of Samuel Johnson's Literary Club, 1764. *Died 4 April 1774.*

PUBLICATIONS

Collections

   *Collected Letters*, edited by Katharine C. Balderston.    1928.
   *Collected Works*, edited by Arthur Friedman.   5 vols., 1966.
   *Poems and Plays*, edited by Tom Davis.    1975.

Plays

   *The Good Natured Man* (produced 1768).    1768.
   *The Grumbler*, from a translation by Charles Sedley of a work of Brueys (produced 1773).    Edited by Alice I. P. Wood, 1931.
   *She Stoops to Conquer; or, The Mistakes of a Night* (produced 1773).    1773; edited by Arthur Friedman, 1968.
   *Threnodia Augustalis, Sacred to the Memory of the Princess Dowager of Wales*, music by Mattia Vento (produced 1772).    1772.
   *The Captivity* (oratorio), in *Miscellaneous Works*.    1820.

Fiction

   *The Vicar of Wakefield*.    1766; edited by Arthur Friedman, 1974.

Verse

*The Traveller; or, A Prospect of Society.*   1764.
*Poems for Young Ladies in Three Parts, Devotional, Moral, and Entertaining.*   1767.
*The Deserted Village.*   1770.
*Retaliation.*   1774.
*The Haunch of Venison: A Poetical Epistle to Lord Clare.*   1776.

Other

*An Enquiry into the Present State of Polite Learning in Europe.*   1759.
*The Bee.*   1759.
*The Mystery Revealed.*   1762.
*The Citizen of the World; or, Letters from a Chinese Philosopher Residing in London to His Friends in the East.*   2 vols., 1762.
*The Life of Richard Nash of Bath.*   1762.
*An History of England in a Series of Letters from a Nobleman to His Son.*   2 vols., 1764.
*An History of the Martyrs and Primitive Fathers of the Church.*   1764.
*Essays.*   1765; revised edition, 1766.
*The Present State of the British Empire in Europe, America, Africa, and Asia.*   1768.
*The Roman History, from the Foundation of the City of Rome to the Destruction of the Western Empire.*   2 vols., 1769; abridged edition, 1772.
*The Life of Thomas Parnell.*   1770.
*The Life of Henry St. John, Lord Viscount Bolingbroke.*   1770.
*The History of England, from the Earliest Times to the Death of George II.*   4 vols., 1771; abridged edition, 1774.
*The Grecian History, from the Earliest State to the Death of Alexander the Great.*   2 vols., 1774.
*An History of the Earth and Animated Nature.*   8 vols., 1774.
*A Survey of Experimental Philosophy, Considered in Its Present State of Improvement.*   2 vols., 1776.

Editor, *The Beauties of English Poesy.*   2 vols., 1767.

Translator, *The Memoirs of a Protestant,* by J. Marteilhe.   2 vols., 1758; edited by A. Dobson, 1895.
Translator, *Plutarch's Lives.*   4 vols., 1762.
Translator, *A Concise History of Philosophy and Philosophers,* by M. Formey.   1766.
Translator, *The Comic Romance of Scarron.*   2 vols., 1775.

Bibliography: *Goldsmith Bibliographically and Biographically Considered* by Temple Scott, 1928.

Reading List: *Goldsmith* by Ralph Wardle, 1957; *Goldsmith* by Clara M. Kirk, 1967; *Goldsmith: A Georgian Study* by Ricardo Quintana, 1967; *Life of Goldsmith* by Henry A. Dobson, 1972; *Goldsmith* by A. Lytton Sells, 1974; *Goldsmith: The Critical Heritage,* edited by George S. Rousseau, 1974; *The Notable Man: The Life and Times of Goldsmith* by John Ginger, 1977.

\*      \*      \*

Oliver Goldsmith's reputation is made up of paradox. His blundering, improvident nature nevertheless won him the loyalty and friendship of figures like Dr. Johnson, Sir Joshua Reynolds, and Edmund Burke. While in society he was a buffoon, his writing testifies to personal charm and an ironic awareness of his own and others' absurdity. Critical opinion of his work similarly varies from acceptance of Goldsmith as the sensitive apologist for past values to appraisal of him as an accomplished social and literary satirist. Indeed, his work can operate on both levels, a fact perhaps recognised by the young Jane Austen in her *Juvenilia* when she took Goldsmith's abridgements of history for young persons as a model for her own exercise in irony.

Drifting into authorship after a mis-spent youth (as Macaulay notes in his disapproving *Life*), Goldsmith turned to hack writing, contributing articles to the *Monthly* and *Critical Reviews* from 1757. His more ambitious *Inquiry into the Present State of Polite Learning* of 1759 won him the reputation of a man of learning and elegant expression. In this last essay he reveals his fundamental dislike of the contemporary cult of sensibility which was to generate not only his own "laughing" form of comedy in the drama but also *The Vicar of Wakefield*. Meeting Smollett, then editor of the *British Magazine*, Goldsmith was encouraged to expand his contributions to literary journalism. He produced the weekly periodical *The Bee*; many papers collected and published in 1765 and 1766 as *Essays*; and, most important, the "Chinese Letters" of 1760–61 collected as *The Citizen of the World*.

The "citizen" is, of course, an Oriental traveller, observing the fashions and foibles of the *bon ton* in London with wide-eyed innocence that carries within it implicit comment and criticism not unmixed with humour. The device was borrowed from the French, notably Montesquieu's *Lettres Persanes* (1721). In each essay the absurdities of behaviour are marked, the whole inter-woven by continuing narratives around the Man in Black, Beau Tibbs, the story of Hingo and Zelis, for instance. In many ways the ironies, improbabilities, and apparent innocence of the Chinese letters prefigure the extended prose romance of *The Vicar of Wakefield*.

This could be seen as Goldsmith's answer to Sterne's *Tristram Shandy* (1759). He had attacked Sterne's sentimental fiction as "obscene and pert" in *The Citizen*; in many ways *The Vicar* parodies Sterne's novel but with such a light hand that it has been taken on face value for many generations as the tale indeed of a family "generous, credulous, simple, and inoffensive." However, Goldsmith early establishes for the observant the manifest danger of complacency in such apparent virtues. His Yorkshire parson displays the moral duplicity of a feeling heart, for Goldsmith's approach to life and art is the opposite of Sterne's relativism and dilettante values.

Goldsmith's moral seriousness (while softened by genial good humour) dominates that other work now considered "classic," *The Deserted Village*. His earlier sortie in the genre of topographical/philosophical verse, *The Traveller*, did much to establish his reputation. It is an accomplished use of convention, where the poet climbs an eminence only to have his mind expanded into contemplation of universal questions. In *The Deserted Village*, however, the poet comes to terms with a particular social problem in a particular landscape as opposed to former abstract musings above imaginary solitudes. "Sweet Auburn" can be identified closely with the village of Nuneham Courtenay, where the local land-owner had recently moved the whole community out in order to extend and improve his landscape park. The fact becomes a catalyst for Goldsmith in a consideration of where aesthetic values and irresponsible wealth lead: a symbol taken from life and not from poetic convention.

Goldsmith's rhymed couplets have grace and ease, particularly when his verse is unlaboured, as in the prologues and epilogues to his own and others' plays. The charm and humour of these can be observed in his later poem *Retaliation*, which has a pointed raciness born out of the settling of personal scores. Always the butt of jokes in the group known as The Club, here he gets his own back with a series of comic epitaphs for the other members. Notable is that for Garrick – "On the stage he was natural, simple, affecting;/Twas only that when he was off he was acting" – but he labels himself the "gooseberry fool."

As a dramatist, Goldsmith exploited both verbal dexterity and the comedy of situation, looking back to Shakespeare in the rejection of the so-called genteel comedy of Hugh Kelly or Richard Cumberland. Affected and strained in tone and action, the drama of sentiment offered to Goldsmith nothing of the "nature and humour" that he saw as the first principle of theatre. However he might despise the sentimental school, he cannot avoid using some of its conventions, the good-natured hero, of course, and the device of paired lovers, but the way these are treated is particular to himself. Together with Sheridan, Goldsmith exploits the theatrical unreality of comedy, using the stage as a separate world of experience with its own laws and therefore demanding the suspension of disbelief in order that farcical unreality might unmask farcical reality. His character Honeydew in *The Good Natured Man* has something in common with Charles Surface in *School for Scandal*, but the tone of Goldsmith's comedy is less brittle than that of Sheridan. This mellow tone, a fundamental wholesomeness, is magnificently encapsulated in *She Stoops to Conquer*.

Goldsmith's first play met with a poor response, as being too "low" in its matter (especially the bailiffs scene), and, though *She Stoops to Conquer* was open to similar criticism, its riotous humour overcame prejudice. In short, it was good theatre and this is testified by its continuing popularity in production. Characters like Tony Lumpkin, Mrs. Hardcastle, and the old Squire have become literary personalities, while the pivot of the plot, Marlow's loss of diffidence in apparently more relaxed circumstances, holds true to human nature. The character of Kate is a liberated heroine in the Shakespearean style, contrasted as in the older comedy with a foil. One is able to relate Goldsmith's "laughing" comedy to that of Shakespeare in many ways, for the Lord of Misrule dominates both.

The range of Goldsmith's work is touched by this same humour and sensitivity, the good heart that is so easily squandered as he himself acknowledged in *The Good Natured Man*, but is just as easily extended with purpose to the reader. As Walter Scott observed, no man contrived "so well to reconcile us to human nature."

—B. C. Oliver-Morden

---

**HILL, Aaron.** English. Born in London, 10 February 1685. Educated at Barnstaple Grammar School, Devon; Westminster School, London. Married Miss Morris in 1710 (died, 1731); nine children. Visited his relative, Lord Paget, then Ambassador in Constantinople, and sent by Paget on a tour of the east, 1700–03; subsequently travelled as a tutor to Sir William Wentworth; settled in London: Manager of the Drury Lane Theatre, 1709–10, and the opera in the Haymarket, 1710–13; managed the Little Theatre, Haymarket, c. 1720–33; Editor, with William Bond, *The Plain-Dealer*, 1724–25; Editor, *The Prompter*, 1734–36; also involved in various unsuccessful business ventures, including extracting oil from beechmast, 1713, colonizing in Georgia, 1718, etc.; retired to Essex, 1738. *Died 8 February 1750.*

PUBLICATIONS

Collections

*Works.* 4 vols., 1753.
*Dramatic Works.* 2 vols., 1760.

Plays

*Elfrid; or, The Fair Inconstant* (produced 1710).   1710; revised version, as *Athelwold*
   (produced 1731), 1732.
*The Walking Statue; or, The Devil in the Wine Cellar* (produced 1710).   With *Elfrid*,
   1710.
*Rinaldo*, music by Handel, from a play by Giacomo Rossi (produced 1711).   1711.
*Il Pastor Fido, The Faithful Shepherd*, music by Handel, from a play by Giacomo Rossi
   (produced 1712).   1712.
*The Fatal Vision; or, The Fall of Siam* (produced 1716).   1716.
*The Fatal Extravagance*, with Joseph Mitchell (produced 1721).   1720; revised version
   (produced 1730), 1726.
*King Henry the Fifth; or, The Conquest of France by the English*, from the play by
   Shakespeare (produced 1723).   1723.
*The Tragedy of Zara*, from a work by Voltaire (produced 1735).   1736.
*Alzira*, from a work by Voltaire (produced 1736).   1736.
*Merope*, from a work by Voltaire (produced 1749).   1749.
*The Roman Revenge*, from a work by Voltaire (produced 1753?).   1753.
*The Insolvent; or, Filial Piety*, from the play *The Guiltless Adultress* by Davenant based
   on *The Fatal Dowry* by Massinger (produced 1758).   1758.
*The Muses in Mourning, Merlin in Love, The Snake in the Grass, Saul*, and *Daraxes*, in
   *Dramatic Works*.   1760.


Verse

*Camillus*.   1707.
*The Invasion: A Poem to the Queen*.   1708.
*The Dedication of the Beech Tree*.   1714.
*The Northern Star*.   1718; revised edition, 1739.
*The Creation: A Pindaric*.   1720.
*The Judgment-Day*.   1721.
*The Progress of Wit: A Caveat*.   1730.
*Advice to the Poets*.   1731.
*The Tears of the Muses*.   1737.
*The Fanciad: An Heroic Poem*.   1743.
*The Impartial: An Address Without Flattery*.   1744.
*The Art of Acting*.   1744.
*Free Thoughts on Faith; or, The Religion of Reason*.   1746.
*Gideon; or, The Patriot: An Epic Poem*.   1749.


Other

*A Full Account of the Present State of the Ottoman Empire*.   1709.
*An Enquiry into the Merit of Assassination*.   1738.
*A Collection of Letters Between Hill, Pope, and Others*.   1751.
*Selections from The Prompter*, edited by W. A. Appleton and K. A. Burnim.   1966.

Editor, *The Plain-Dealer* (periodical).   2 vols., 1730.

Translator, with Nahum Tate, *The Celebrated Speeches of Ajax and Ulysses*, by
   Ovid.   1708.

Reading List: *The Life and Works of Hill* by H. Ludwig, 1911; *Hill, Poet, Dramatist, Projector* by Dorothy Brewster, 1913.

          *     *     *

Aaron Hill was a man of great ambition but very frequently a loser. As a teenager he visited Constantinople (where a relative, Lord Paget, was British ambassador) but his book on the Ottoman Empire was written too early in life and later he deprecated it. He addressed a poem to Lord Peterborough but failed to take the preferment it occasioned. He wrote another in honor of Peter the Great and was awarded a gold medal – which he never collected. He proposed the colonization of Georgia but then dropped the idea. He invented some gadgets and processes – he patented one for extracting oil from beechmast – but nothing came of it. He wrote the libretto for Handel's *Rinaldo* (1711) but did not benefit either from the subsequent popularity for opera or from the spate of parodies, ballad operas, and other reactions which followed the Italian fad. He was appointed by William Collier to manage the Theatre Royal in Drury Lane but the actors beat him up and rioted: for this Powell was dismissed and Booth, Bickerstaff, Keen and Leigh disciplined, but in the end Hill suffered most. He defended Shakespeare against the attacks of Voltaire when the French genius was temporarily touted over the native one and said some nasty things about Pope in *The Progress of Wit*, which gained him the notoriety of a mention in *The Dunciad*. He adapted several of Voltaire's plays for the English stage but Arthur Murphy rather upstaged him with *The Orphan of China* (1759). His version of Voltaire's *Merope* was commanded as a benefit performance by Frederick, Prince of Wales – but Hill died the night before the performance.

As a playwright, Hill was not notable, though his early farce *The Walking Statue* showed more promise than such poems as *Camillus* and *The Northern Star*. *Elfrid; or, The Fair Inconstant* betrayed some of the jejune quality in *A Full Account of the Ottoman Empire*, and, while rhodomontade might pass on the stage, when *Aethelwold* (the revised version of *Elfrid*) appeared in print it was greeted with well-deserved ridicule. I must confess that Voltaire's pseudo-classical plays leave me cold and that Hill's English *réchauffages* are no help. Even the poetry of Stephen Duck (1705–1756) is probably better than Hill's if one must have a Wiltshire bard of the time, though Hill retired to family farms in Wiltshire after London rejected him, while Duck committed suicide after his brief vogue. Hill's verse is more pompous than that of John Home's *Douglas* (1757) but far less impressive, and Hill's greatest contribution to poetry was (when he was self-importantly setting himself up as *censor elegantarium* in competition with Pope) in recognizing true talent in James Thomson's *Winter* (1726, brought to Hill's attention by Thomson's friend David Mallet) and generously publicizing it. One might add that Hill regarded Thomson's *Liberty* as "mighty work" and "the last stretched blaze of our expiring genius" – probably because Thomson was then the heir-apparent to Pope. In his controversy with Pope, Hill was lively but did not really emerge as well as Colley Cibber. In the end he made up with Pope and numbered him and Richardson and many other celebrities among his friends. He befriended Richard Savage and wrote about him in his newspaper.

It was his journalism and his letters that saved Hill from being "a bit of a bore." *The Plain-Dealer* (23 March 1724 to 7 May 1725), conducted with William Bond, "maintained a good philosophic literary level" (Bonamy Dobrée, *English Literature in the Early Eighteenth Century*, 1959), and *The Prompter* (12 November 1734 to 2 July 1736) is of interest to all students of the theatre, its 173 numbers full of good criticism. Moreover Hill's letters are "always in the centre of the literary scene" (Dobrée) and concern Pope and *The Dunciad*; projects involving real estate and potash; coffee, sugar, and the tax on Madeira; Drury Lane and actors like Barton Booth and Robert Wilks; an ill-fated attempt to run the opera at the Haymarket; advice to Thomson on the use of capitals and to actors about tone and delivery; a letter to Sir Robert Walpole on "the encouragement of able *writers*" and one to Lady Walpole on rock-gardens; praise of Richardson's *Pamela* and criticism of Mallet's *Euridice*;

communications to celebrities as different as Peterborough and Voltaire. Perhaps Hill was, as Pope waspishly said, a "bad author" but he was a fascinating individual, and the letters do much to prove the truth of another judgment of the Wasp of Twickenham: that Aaron Hill was "not quite a swan, not wholly a goose." If only as the author of *The Prompter*, Hill deserves a more modern study than those of Brewster or Ludwig.

—Leonard R.N. Ashley

---

**HOLCROFT, Thomas.** English. Born in London, 10 December 1745. Self-educated. Married four times, lastly to Louisa Mercier; one son and two daughters. Worked as a stableboy in Newmarket, Suffolk, 1757–60, and in his father's cobbler's stall, London, 1761–64; taught school in Liverpool, 1764; resumed his trade of shoemaker, London, 1764–69, and contributed to the *Whitehall Evening Post*; tutor in the family of Granville Sharp, 1769; prompter at a Dublin theatre, 1770–71; strolling player in the provinces in England, 1771–78; returned to London, 1778, and thereafter a prolific writer: contributed to the *Westminster Magazine*, *Wit's Magazine*, *Town and Country*, and early numbers of the *English Review*; actor and playwright at Drury Lane Theatre, 1778–84; Correspondent in Paris for the *Morning Herald*, 1783; joined the Society for Constitutional Information, 1792: indicted for treason, imprisoned, then discharged, 1794; moved to Hamburg, 1799, and tried, unsuccessfully, to establish the *European Repository*; lived in Paris, 1801–03, then returned to London: set up a printing business with his brother-in-law, 1803, which subsequently failed. *Died 23 March 1809.*

PUBLICATIONS

Plays

> *The Crisis; or, Love and Fear* (produced 1778).
> *Duplicity* (produced 1781).    1781; as *The Masked Friend* (produced 1796).
> *The Noble Peasant*, music by William Shield (produced 1784).    1784.
> *The Follies of a Day; or, The Marriage of Figaro*, from a play by Beaumarchais (produced 1784).    1785; revised version, 1881; revised version, from the opera by da Ponte, music by Mozart (produced 1819), 1819.
> *The Choleric Fathers*, music by William Shield (produced 1785).    1785.
> *Sacred Dramas Written in French by la Comtesse de Genlis.*    1785.
> *Seduction* (produced 1787).    1787.
> *The School for Arrogance*, from a play by Destouches (produced 1791).    1791.
> *The Road to Ruin* (produced 1792).    1792; edited by Ruth I. Aldrich, 1968.
> *Love's Frailties* (produced 1794).    1794.
> *Heigh-Ho! for a Husband.*    1794.
> *The Rival Queens; or, Drury Lane and Covent Garden* (produced 1794).
> *The Deserted Daughter*, from a work by Diderot (produced 1795).    1795.
> *The Man of Ten Thousand* (produced 1796).    1796.
> *The Force of Ridicule* (produced 1796).
> *Knave or Not?*, from plays by Goldoni (produced 1798).    1798.
> *He's Much to Blame* (produced 1798).    1798.

*The Inquisitor* (produced 1798).   1798.

*The Old Clothesman*, music by Thomas Attwood (produced 1799).   Songs published 1799(?).

*Deaf and Dumb; or, The Orphan Protected*, from a play by de Bouilly (produced 1801).   1801.

*The Escapes; or, The Water-Carrier*, music by Thomas Attwood, songs by T. J. Dibdin, from an opera by J. N. Nouilly, music by Cherubini (produced 1801).

*A Tale of Mystery*, from a play by Pixérécourt (produced 1802).   1802.

*Hear Both Sides* (produced 1803).   1803.

*The Lady of the Rock* (produced 1805).   1805.

*The Vindictive Man* (produced 1806).   1806.


Fiction

*Alwyn; or, The Gentleman Comedian*, with William Nicholson.   1780.

*The Family Picture; or, Domestic Dialogues on Amiable Subjects.*   1783.

*An Amorous Tale of the Chaste Loves of Peter the Long and His Most Honoured Friend Dame Blanche Bazu.*   1786.

*Anna St. Ives.*   1792; edited by Peter Faulkner, 1970.

*The Adventures of Hugh Trevor.*   1794; edited by Seamus Deane, 1973.

*Memoirs of Bryan Perdue.*   1805.


Verse

*Elegies.*   1777.

*Human Happiness; or, The Sceptic.*   1783.

*Tales in Verse, Critical, Satirical, Humorous.*   1806.


Other

*A Plain and Succinct Narrative of the Late [Gordon] Riots.*   1780; edited by Garland Garvey Smith, 1944.

*The Trial of the Hon. George Gordon.*   1781.

*Memoirs of Baron de Tott, Containing the State of the Turkish Empire and the Crimea.*   2 vols., 1785.

*The Secret History of the Court of Berlin.*   2 vols., 1789.

*A Narrative of Facts Relating to a Prosecution for High Treason.*   2 vols., 1795.

*A Letter to William Windham on the Intemperance and Danger of His Public Conduct.*   1795.

*Travels from Hamburg Through Westphalia, Holland, and the Netherlands.*   2 vols., 1804.

*Memoirs*, completed by William Hazlitt.   3 vols., 1816; edited by Elbridge Colby, as *The Life of Holcroft*, 2 vols., 1925.

Editor, *Letter on Egypt*, by Mr. Savary.   2 vols., 1786.

Editor, and Translator, *Posthumous Works of Frederick, King of Prussia.*   13 vols., 1789.

Editor, *The Theatrical Recorder.*   2 vols., 1805–06.

Translator, *Philosophical Essays with Observations on the Laws and Customs of Several Eastern Nations*, by Foucher d'Osbornville.   1784.

Translator, *Tales of the Castle*, by la Comtesse de Genlis. 5 vols., 1785.

Translator, *Caroline of Lichtfield*, by Baroness de Montolieu. 2 vols., 1786.

Translator, *Historical and Critical Memoirs of the Life and Writings of Voltaire*, by Chaudon. 1786.

Translator, *The Present State of the Empire of Morocco*, by Chenier. 2 vols., 1788.

Translator, *The Life of Baron Frederick Trenck.* 3 vols., 1788.

Translator, *Essays on Physiognomy*, by J. C. Lavater. 3 vols., 1789.

Translator, *Travels Through Germany, Switzerland, and Italy*, by Frederick Leopold, Count Stolberg. 2 vols., 1796–97.

Translator, *Herman and Dorothea*, by Goethe. 1801.


Bibliography: *A Bibliography of Holcroft* by Elbridge Colby, 1922.

Reading List: *Holcroft and the Revolutionary Novel* by Rodney M. Baine, 1965; *The English Jacobin Novel* by Gary Kelly, 1976.

\*      \*      \*

Thomas Holcroft was a self-taught man of letters, and one of the leading radical writers of the period of the French Revolution. His early writing was mostly for the theatre, and both *The School for Arrogance* and *The Road to Ruin* were successful in combining sentimental melodrama with the new philosophy. But with changing theatrical taste, Holcroft's plays passed into an oblivion from which they are yet to be restored. He chose to use the novel form for the fuller exposition of his political outlook, an outlook clearly influenced by his friendship with William Godwin, the most famous radical intellectual of the day, and his acquaintance with other radicals like Tom Paine and Mary Wollstonecraft.

Holcroft's two major novels are *Anna St. Ives* and *The Adventures of Hugh Trevor*. *Anna St. Ives* may be regarded as the equivalent in fiction of Godwin's *Political Justice*. It expresses its criticism of society through the contrasting contenders for the hand of the heroine, Anna: the rationalist Frank Henley, the virtuous son of the steward of Anna's father, and the aristocratic rake Coke Clifton. Clifton is a character in the line of Richardson's Lovelace in *Clarissa*, confident, witty, and unprincipled. He is allowed to express himself with a theatrical exuberance which gives the novel some vitality: "Should I be obliged to come like Jove to Semele, in flames, and should we both be reduced to ashes in the conflict, I will enjoy her!" However, the novel has a clear doctrinaire intention, which results in the defeat of Clifton and the marriage of Frank and Anna. The extravagance of Holcroft's idealism comes out in the final conversion of Clifton himself to the high-minded radicalism of his two unfailing friends.

*Hugh Trevor* is less diagrammatic in its rendering of life, but no less didactic in intention. The story of Trevor's life is basically picaresque, with a variety of adventures and events, but the moral of his experiences is clear: society is corrupt, and reason must guide the individual if he is to avoid its coercions. But there is also some psychological development, which would seem to have an autobiographical origin, in Trevor's gradual development of control over his original impulsiveness. When this is allied with a vigorous satirical attack on various aspects of society, including the Church, the law and reactionary politicians, the overall effect is a novel of considerable interest. Together with *Anna*, it justifies Holcroft's claim to be considered as a significant participant in an important tradition of rationalist social idealism.

—Peter Faulkner

**HOME, John.** Scottish. Born in Leith, near Edinburgh, 21 September 1722. Educated at the grammar school in Leith; University of Edinburgh, graduated 1742. Fought on the Hanoverian side in the Edinburgh volunteers, subsequently as a Lieutenant in the Glasgow volunteers, 1745–46: taken prisoner at Falkirk, 1746. Married Mary Home in 1770. Licensed to preach by the presbytery of Edinburgh, 1745; Minister of Athelstaneford, East Lothian, 1747 until he resigned before he could be tried on charges of profanity in his play *Douglas*, 1757; Private Secretary to the Earl of Bute, and subsequently tutor to the Prince of Wales, from 1757: granted pension by George III on his accession, 1760; Conservator of Scots privileges at Campvere, Holland, from 1763; built a mansion in Kilduff, East Lothian, and lived there, 1770–79; settled in Edinburgh, 1779. *Died 5 September 1808.*

PUBLICATIONS

Collections

*Works.*   3 vols., 1822.

Plays

*Douglas* (produced 1756).   1757; edited by Gerald D. Parker, 1972.
*Agis,* music by William Boyce (produced 1758).   1758.
*The Siege of Aquileia* (produced 1760).   1760.
*Dramatic Works.*   1760; revised edition, 2 vols., 1798.
*The Fatal Discovery* (produced 1769).   1769.
*Alonzo* (produced 1773).   1773.
*Alfred* (produced 1778).   1778.

Other

*The History of the Rebellion in the Year 1745.*   1802.

Reading List: *The Works of Home* by Henry Mackenzie, 1822; *Home: A Study of His Life and Works* by Alice E. Gipson, 1917.

*       *       *

Although John Home wrote six tragedies, his reputation is based almost entirely on *Douglas,* the second of his plays in order of composition but the first to be performed. After Garrick declined the play at Drury Lane, *Douglas* was performed with great success in Edinburgh, which led to a remarkably heated controversy concerned chiefly with the impropriety of a minister contributing to "wicked" theatrical activity. *Douglas* was also an immediate success when performed at Covent Garden in London, quickly became standard repertory fare, and remained popular for over a century.

One of the eighteenth century's best blank-verse tragedies, *Douglas* deals with the untimely death of the valiant Douglas and the ensuing suicide of his mother, Lady Randolph, with whom he has been reunited after having been separated since infancy. The contrast between

Lady Randolph's past suffering and current, though temporary, joy is central to the play, which seeks to evoke "celestial melancholy" by focusing on tragic irony and pity for Lady Randolph's frustrated maternal love. The play's popularity can also be attributed to its fervid language, highly romantic setting, and appeal to Scottish national pride.

Of Home's five other plays, *Agis*, *The Siege of Aquileia*, *The Fatal Discovery*, and *Alonzo* were moderately well-received on the eighteenth-century stage, while his last effort, *Alfred*, ran for only three nights. With the exception of *The Siege of Aquileia*, these plays also employ tragic irony, melancholy atmospheres, or romantic settings to evoke pathos, but are generally inferior to *Douglas*.

*Agis*, written before *Douglas*, deals with the assassination of a political hero who fails to recognize the treachery of his enemies. In *The Fatal Discovery*, based on one of James Macpherson's Ossianic fragments, the heroine, Rivine, commits suicide after placing love above personal honor. Rivine is made to appear an innocent victim of deception; hence emphasis is placed on the growing pathos of her situation as the play progresses. *Alonzo* is nearly identical to *Douglas* in plot conception and in stressing frustrated maternal affection; however, Lady Randolph's suicide is well-motivated and moving, whereas Ormisinda, in *Alonzo*, kills herself for no apparent reason at the moment when various misunderstandings could be corrected and disaster averted. *Alfred* is a melodrama that deserves to remain the most obscure of Home's plays. It consists of a series of schemes devised by Alfred to save his betrothed from Hinguar, the Danish king.

The best of these five plays is *The Siege of Aquileia*, in which Aemilius, a Roman consul and governor, must either sacrifice his sons or betray his country and personal honor. Home handles Aemilius's dilemma effectively, making the choice progressively more difficult. This is the only one of Home's plays in which the protagonist must choose between equally worthy, conflicting sets of values; hence it allows for more complex tragic effects than the pathos that remains uppermost in all of Home's other plays.

—James S. Malek

---

**HOWARD, Sir Robert.**   English.   Born in England in 1626; son of the Earl of Berkshire; brother-in-law of John Dryden, *q.v.* Probably educated at Magdalen College, Oxford. Married 1) Ann Kingsmill in 1645, one daughter; 2) Lady Honora O'Brien in 1665, one son; 3) Annabella Dives in 1692. Royalist: knighted for bravery at the second battle of Newbury, 1644; imprisoned during the Commonwealth at Windsor Castle; after the Restoration became Member of Parliament for Stockbridge, Hampshire, was made a Knight of the Bath, and became Secretary to the Commissioners of the Treasury; Auditor of the Exchequer, 1677 until his death; Member of Parliament for Castle Rising, Norfolk, 1678–98; Privy Councillor, 1688; commissioner to enquire into the state of the fleet, 1690; commander of the militia horse, 1690. *Died 3 September 1698.*

PUBLICATIONS

Plays

*The Blind Lady,* in *Poems.*   1660.
*The Surprisal* (produced 1662).   In *Four New Plays,* 1665.

The Committee; or, The Faithful Irishman (produced 1662). In Four New Plays, 1665; edited by Carryl N. Thurber, 1921.

The Indian Queen (produced 1664). In Four New Plays, 1665; revised version, music by Purcell (produced 1695); in Works 8 by Dryden, 1962.

The Vestal Virgin; or, The Roman Ladies (produced 1665). In Four New Plays, 1665.

Four New Plays. 1665; expanded edition, as Five New Plays, 1692; as Dramatic Works, 1722.

The Great Favourite; or, The Duke of Lerma (produced 1668). 1668; edited by D. D. Arundell, in Dryden and Howard, 1929.

The Country Gentleman, with George Villiers, edited by Arthur H. Scouten and Robert D. Hume. 1976.


Verse

Poems. 1660.
The Duel of the Stags. 1668.


Other

An Account of the State of His Majesty's Revenue. 1680.
The Life and Reign of King Richard the Second. 1680.
Historical Observations upon the Reigns of Edward I, II, III, and Richard II. 1689.
A Letter to Mr. Samuel Johnson. 1692.
The History of Religion. 1694; as An Account of the Growth of Deism, 1709.


Reading List: Howard: A Critical Biography by Harold J. Oliver, 1963 (includes bibliography).

*     *     *

Sir Robert Howard was active in various aspects of the revival of drama upon the re-opening of the theatres in 1660, as he not only wrote comedies and one of the earliest heroic plays but also engaged in dramatic theory. A new kind of tragedy was emerging, and Harold J. Oliver calls Howard's first play, The Blind Lady, "half-way between Jacobean tragedy and Heroic drama." Howard then went all the way towards creating a new form in The Indian Queen. Here we find an epic hero, a conflict between the claims of Love and Honour, serious debates, and spectacular stage effects. The reception of this new type of drama led Howard into unprofitable literary controversies over the place of rhymed verse in tragedy and the validity of tragi-comedy.

Of his four comedies, The Committee was his great success, holding the stage into the nineteenth century. This vivacious work presents an implacable conflict between the puritans and the royalists toward the end of the Commonwealth period and contains an intrinsically comic figure in the Irish servant Teague. More important, however, in a critical analysis of Howard as a playwright is his achieving what strikes the reader as a genuine rather than an artificial portrayal of women in his imaginative creation of the heroine Ruth and the villain Mrs. Day, a former dairy maid who has risen to become the wife of the chairman of the sequestration committee. These two women are more than a match for the men throughout the play.

Similar psychological insight and emphasis on the role of women appear in The Country Gentleman, the long-lost political comedy by Howard and George Villiers, which was discovered in 1973. In the play, Howard experiments with the love game between the romantic couples, a technique which was to become standard practice in later sex-comedies of the Restoration. Yet Howard proceeds with sturdy independence to present an exemplary father (unheard of in this early period), to champion the country against the city, and to engage in satire which includes positive as well as negative examples. His neoclassical taste is revealed in the structure of this comedy, all of which is set in two rooms of one house, with the time of the action only slightly exceeding the actual time of the representation.

After a promising beginning as a playwright, Howard abandoned literature and turned to a full career in politics.

—Arthur H. Scouten

HUGHES, John.  English.   Born in Marlborough, Wiltshire, 29 January 1677; brother of the translator Jabez Hughes. Educated at a dissenting academy, probably in Little Britain, London. Worked in the Ordnance Office, London, and served as Secretary to various commissions for the purchase of lands for the royal dockyards; Secretary to the commissions of peace in the court of chancery, from 1717. *Died 17 February 1720.*

PUBLICATIONS

Collections

*Poems on Several Occasions, with Some Select Essays,* edited by W. Duncombe.   2 vols., 1735.

Plays

*Six Cantatas,* music by J. C. Pepusch (produced 1710).   1710.
*Calypso and Telemachus,* music by J. E. Galliard (produced 1712).   1712.
*Apollo and Daphne: A Masque,* music by J. C. Pepusch (produced 1716).   1716.
*Orestes.*   1717.
*The Siege of Damascus* (produced 1720).   1720.

Verse

*The Triumph of Peace.*   1698.
*The Court of Neptune.*   1699.
*The House of Nassau: A Pindaric Ode.*   1702.
*An Ode in Praise of Music.*   1703.
*An Ode to the Creator of the World, Occasioned by the Fragments of Orpheus.*   1713.
*An Ode for the Birthday of the Princess of Wales.*   1716.
*The Ecstasy: An Ode.*   1720.

Other

*A Review of the Case of Ephraim and Judah.*   1705.
*The Lay-Monastery, Consisting of Essays, Discourses, etc.,* with Richard Blackmore.   1714.
*A Layman's Thoughts on the Late Treatment of the Bishop of Bangor.*   1717.
*Charon; or, The Ferry-Boat: A Vision.*   1719.
*The Complicated Guilt of the Late Rebellion.*   1745.
*Letters of Several Eminent Persons Deceased,* with others, edited by J. Duncombe.   1772; as *The Correspondence of Hughes and Several of His Friends,* 2 vols., 1773.

Editor, *A Complete History of England,* vols. 1–2, by W. Kennett.   1706.
Editor, *Advice from Parnassus,* by Traiano Boccalini.   1706.
Editor, *The Works of Spenser.*   6 vols., 1715; commentary edited by Scott Elledge, in *Eighteenth-Century Critical Essays,* vol. 1, 1961.

Translator, *Fontenelle's Dialogues of the Dead, with Two Original Dialogues.*   1708.
Translator, *The History of the Revolutions in Portugal,* by the Abbot de Vertot.   1712.
Translator, *Letters of Abelard and Heloise, Extracted Chiefly from Bayle.*   1718 (3rd edition).

Reading List: "Some Sources for *The Siege of Damascus*" by John R. Moore, in *Huntington Library Quarterly 21,* 1958.

\*        \*        \*

Critics have been reluctant to pass favourable judgment on John Hughes. Eminent contemporaries were less than generous towards his achievement, and Johnson's *Life* is non-committal. Gibbon, on the other hand, praised *The Siege of Damascus* for its "rare merit of blending nature and history...." As a playwright Hughes had some success in the sphere of high tragedy; but his more ambitious poems such as *The House of Nassau* and the *Ode to the Creator of the World* lack coherence, while his shorter verses are overburdened with Augustan conventionalities. What redeems Hughes's considerable talent is his excellent understanding of other authors' intentions (as in the "Essay on Allegorical Poetry" prefixed to his 1715 edition of Spenser) and his discerning views on the potentialities of sung poetry.

At a time when Italian vocal music was all the rage, Hughes aimed "to improve a sort of (English) verse, in regular measures, purposely fitted for music ... which, of all the modern kinds, seems to be the only one that can now properly be called lyrics." Rejecting Edmund Waller's notion that "soft words with nothing in them make a song" and paying due respect to the composer's demand for a congenial text, Hughes produced *Six Cantatas* (set by J. C. Pepusch) and other brief works in which the airs and recitatives employ suitably contrasting accentuations. On a more ambitious scale are several odes, also intended for music. The inventiveness they display is again evident in stage masques written as an alternative genre to Italianate music drama. A more resourceful composer than Pepusch might have created a minor masterpiece out of *Apollo and Daphne*; for his opera *Calypso and Telemachus* Hughes had collaborated with J. E. Galliard, for whose music Handel had a high regard. This work constituted an attempt to refute "a late Opinion among some, that *English* words are not proper for Musick" and bears out Hughes's contention that the alleged shortcomings of the English language need not deter an inventive librettist.

Hughes's prose writings include translations and periodical essays. His work as a whole reveals a wide knowledge of general literature; although overshadowed by Steele, Addison, and Pope his critical abilities place him well above the level of incorrigible mediocrity.

—E. D. Mackerness

---

**INCHBALD, Elizabeth (née Simpson).**    English.    Born in Stanningfield, near Bury St. Edmunds, Suffolk, 15 October 1753. Married the actor and painter Joseph Inchbald in 1772 (died, 1779). Settled in London, 1772; debut as an actress, playing opposite her husband, Bristol, 1772; subsequently appeared in various Scottish towns, 1772–76, various English towns, 1776–78, and under Tate Wilkinson in Yorkshire, 1778–80; appeared on the London stage, 1780 until her retirement, 1789. *Died 1 August 1821.*

PUBLICATIONS

Plays

A Mogul Tale; or, The Descent of the Balloon (produced 1784).    1788.
I'll Tell You What (produced 1785).    1786.
Appearance Is Against Them (produced 1785).    1785.
The Widow's Vow, from a play by Patrat (produced 1786).    1786.
Such Things Are (produced 1787).    1788.
The Midnight Hour; or, War of Wits, from a play by Dumaniant (produced 1787).    1787.
All on a Summer's Day (produced 1787).
Animal Magnetism (produced 1788).    1788(?).
The Child of Nature, from a play by Mme. de Genlis (produced 1788).    1788.
The Married Man, from a play by Philippe Néricault-Destouches (produced 1789).    1789.
The Hue and Cry, from a play by Dumaniant (produced 1791).
Next Door Neighbours, from plays by L. S. Mercier and Philippe Néricault-Destouches (produced 1791).    1791.
Young Men and Old Women, from a play by Gresset (produced 1792).
Every One Has His Fault (produced 1793).    1792; edited by Allardyce Nicoll in *Lesser English Comedies of the Eighteenth Century,* 1931.
The Wedding Day (produced 1794).    1794.
Wives as They Were and Maids as They Are (produced 1797).    1797.
Lovers' Vows, from a play by Kotzebue (produced 1798).    1798.
The Wise Men of the East, from a play by Kotzebue (produced 1799).    1799.
To Marry, or Not to Marry (produced 1805).    1805.
The Massacre and A Case of Conscience, in *Memoirs of Mrs. Inchbald* by James Boaden.    2 vols., 1833.

Fiction

*A Simple Story* 1791; edited by J. M. S. Tompkins, 1967.
*Nature and Art* 1796; edited by W. B. Scott, 1886.

Other

Editor, *The British Theatre; or, A Collection of Plays with Biographical and Critical Remarks.* 25 vols., 1808.
Editor, *A Collection of Farces and Other Afterpieces.* 7 vols., 1809.
Editor, *The Modern Theatre.* 10 vols., 1809.

Bibliography: "An Inchbald Bibliography" by George L. Joughlin, in *Studies in English,* 1934.

Reading List: *Memoirs of Mrs. Inchbald* by James Boaden, 2 vols., 1833; *Inchbald and Her Circle* by Samuel R. Littlewood, 1921; *Inchbald, Novelist* by William MacKee, 1935; *Inchbald et la Comédie "Sentimentale" Anglaise au XVIII Siècle* by Françoise Moreux, 1971.

\*       \*       \*

"Now Mrs. Inchbald was all heart," said James Boaden, her biographer, and the statement is as true of her writings as of her life. It is not the whole truth, of course; Boaden's memoir bears ample evidence of her independent spirit, her chasteness of mind and morals, her political liberalism, her candour, and her ardent and life-long pursuit of intellectual self-improvement. These too went to shape her plays and novels. Her plays reveal a fairly constant moral interest, combined with concern for domestic virtues set against the temptations of fashionable society, and working on the conventions of sentimental comedy and the social, scientific, religious, political, and literary topics of the day. She kept well abreast of changing theatrical tastes in the last two decades of the century, but constantly strove to give her slender subjects, complicated plots, and conventional characters some serious moral content. So, as the writer of an epilogue to one of her adaptations from French put it, her version had "the merit/Of giving Gallic Froth – true BRITISH SPIRIT." Her dramas, even those taken from French or German originals (such as Kotzebue's *Lovers' Vows*), were made her own not so much by their themes or techniques as by her thorough subordination of her borrowed materials to her personal version of the moral and aesthetic values of the time. As J. Taylor put it in his prologue to her last play, *To Marry or Not to Marry*, "In all, her anxious hope was still to find,/Some useful moral for the feeling mind."

Her novels were her real achievement, however, and to them she devoted the painstaking care of the conscious artist. These fictions carry many of the same themes and techniques as her plays, and her skill at stagecraft is everywhere apparent in dialogue and the management of scenes, but what she adds in her novels to the technical proficiency of the experienced playwright is an acutely observed sentimental realism. For in both her novels, but especially in the first, *A Simple Story*, can be felt the pressure of autobiography, of the many hours the young woman, wife, and widow had devoted not just to study, but to reflection, and to the practice of that candour which was self-knowledge. From her knowledge of herself, combined with her varied social experience, and informed by her reading in moral writers of all kinds, came that authenticity of psychological observation which made her novels so admired by the likes of William Godwin and Maria Edgeworth. For her, as for so many of the women writers of her day, moral education, the chastening of sensibility by experience, reflection, reason, and reading, was the basic form to be sought in life. In her first novel this form is given all the symmetry, deployed through parallels and contrasts in plot, character, and incident, that could be expected from a kind, even a fictitious kind, of moral discourse. In her second novel, moral education is made more of a public issue, diffused into a satire on the institutions of society, but still shaped by the kind of antithesis represented by the novel's title, *Nature and Art*. Autobiography and moral and social issues are not separate in her novels, then, but fused successfully in fictional form. It was this achievement that won her novels admiration in her own day, and makes them still worth reading now.

—Gary Kelly

---

**KELLY, Hugh.**   Irish.   Born in Killarney in 1739. Received very little formal education; apprenticed to a staymaker. Married in 1761; had five children. Moved to London, 1760, and worked as a staymaker and attorney's copying-clerk, and as writer for one of the daily papers; subsequently Editor of the *Court Magazine* and of the *Lady's Museum* from 1761; also wrote political pamphlets for the bookseller Pottinger, contributed series of essays "The Babler" to Owen's *Weekly Chronicle*, edited the *Public Ledger*, and gained a reputation as a theatrical critic; began to write for the theatre, 1768; employed as a writer by the government from c. 1770, and subsequently received a pension from Lord North; studied law, called to the Bar, Middle Temple, London, 1774, and gave up writing to practise law at the Old Bailey and Middlesex sessions. *Died 3 February 1777.*

PUBLICATIONS

Plays

    *L'Amour A-la-Mode; or, Love-a-la-Mode.*   1760.
    *False Delicacy* (produced 1768).   1768.
    *A Word to the Wise* (produced 1770).   1770.
    *Clementina* (produced 1771).   1771.
    *The School for Wives,* with William Addington, from a play by Molière (produced 1773).   1774.
    *The Romance of an Hour,* from a story by J. F. Marmontel (produced 1774).   1774.
    *The Man of Reason* (produced 1776).

Fiction

    *Memoirs of a Magdalen; or, The History of Louisa Mildmay.*   1767.

Verse

    *An Elegy to the Memory of the Earl of Bath.*   1765 (2nd edition).
    *Thespis; or, A Critical Examination into the Merits of All the Principal Performers Belonging to Drury Lane Theatre.*   1766; revised edition, 1766; part 2, 1767.

Other

*The Babler.*    2 vols., 1767.
*Works.*    1778.

Reading List: "Kelly: His Place in the Sentimental School" by Mark Schorer, in *Philological Quarterly,* 1933; "Some Remarks on 18th Century Delicacy, with a Note on Kelly's *False Delicacy*" by C. J. Rawson, in *Journal of English and Germanic Philology 61,* 1962.

\*        \*        \*

Hugh Kelly typifies the mid-eighteenth-century Grub-Street hack: he edited two magazines, the *Lady's Museum* and the *Court Magazine,* and contributed essays and poetic ephemerae to others. His sentimental novel, *Memoirs of a Magdalen: or, The History of Louisa Mildmay,* appeared first in Owen's *Weekly Chronicle,* as did his series of essays *The Babler* (1763–1766). He wrote pro-government pieces for, and edited, *The Public Ledger* for which the administration rewarded him with a £200 pension – but he died poor. Imitating Charles Churchill's poetic satire on the theatres, *The Rosciad,* Kelly wrote *Thespis,* the two parts of which delineated the actors and writers of Drury Lane and of Covent Garden. Having criticized the contemporary theatre, Kelly then wrote *False Delicacy* for Drury Lane, a comedy that Johnson characterized as "totally void of character," but which outplayed Covent Garden's offering, Goldsmith's *Good Natur'd Man.* Critics have increasingly suggested that the work is less a sentimantal comedy than a mildly witty reproof of delicacy. At each of the two performances of Kelly's second produced comedy, *A Word to the Wise,* Kelly's friends and supporters of Wilkes, who were paying Kelly back for being a ministry writer, caused near riots. (In 1777, to benefit Kelly's widow and six children, Johnson wrote a prologue to this comedy for a performance at Covent Garden.)

Kelly's next play, the verse tragedy *Clementina,* was brought out anonymously, and though it lasted nine performances it has no merit: a contemporary reported, "A man can't hiss and yawn at the same time." *The School for Wives,* however, at first ascribed for protection to Captain William Addington, received good printed reviews, as did Kelly's afterpiece, *The Romance of an Hour,* adapted from Marmontel's tale *L' Amitié à l'épreuve. The Man of Reason,* Kelly's final comedy, lasted one performance.

Essays in *The Babler,* and the comedies *False Delicacy, A Word to the Wise,* and *A School for Wives,* offer the Horatian precept that art must morally instruct (and possibly therefore ennoble) as it entertains. *Thespis* is important as a gossip's recounting of Drury Lane and Covent Garden performers. Neither of Kelly's best plays, *False Delicacy* and *A School for Wives,* seems likely to be revived, but they provided good acting roles which sport with the conventions of sentimentality and are graceful theatrical properties.

—Peter A. Tasch

---

**LEE, Nathaniel.**   English.   Born in Hatfield, Hertfordshire, probably in 1653. Educated at Westminster School, London; Trinity College, Cambridge, 1665–68, B.A. 1668. Settled in London, and at first attempted to become an actor; abandoned acting for writing for the stage c. 1672; a friend of Rochester and his circle: led a dissolute life, and undermined his health and reason by drinking: confined in Bethlehem Hospital (Bedlam), 1684–89. *Died* (buried) *6 May 1692.*

PUBLICATIONS

Collections

*Works,* edited by Thomas B. Stroup and Arthur L. Cooke.    2 vols., 1954–55.

Plays

*Nero, Emperor of Rome* (produced 1674).    1675.
*Sophonisba; or, Hannibal's Overthrow* (produced 1675).    1675; edited by Bonamy Dobrée, in *Five Heroic Plays,* 1960.
*Gloriana; or, The Court of Augustus Caesar* (produced 1676).    1676.
*The Rival Queens; or, The Death of Alexander the Great* (produced 1677).    1677; edited by Paul F. Vernon, 1970.
*Oedipus,* with Dryden (produced 1678).    1679.
*Mithridates, King of Pontus* (produced 1678).    1678.
*Caesar Borgia, The Son of Pope Alexander the Sixth* (produced 1679).    1679.
*Lucius Junius Brutus, Father of His Country* (produced 1680).    1681; edited by John Loftis, 1967.
*Theodosius; or, The Force of Love* (produced 1680).    1680.
*The Princess of Cleve,* from a novel by Mme. de la Fayette (produced 1681).    1689.
*The Duke of Guise,* with Dryden (produced 1682).    1683.
*Constantine the Great* (produced 1683).    1684.
*The Massacre of Paris* (produced 1689).    1689.

Verse

*To the Prince and Princess of Orange upon Their Marriage.*    1677.
*To the Duke on His Return.*    1682.
*On the Death of Mrs. Behn.*    1689.
*On Their Majesties' Coronation.*    1689.

Bibliography: by A. L. McLeod, in *Restoration and 18th-Century Theatre Research 1,* 1962.

Reading List: *Otway and Lee* by Roswell G. Ham, 1931; "The Satiric Design of Lee's *The Princess of Cleve*" by Robert D. Hume, in *Journal of English and Germanic Philology,* 1976.

*      *      *

Nathaniel Lee was the most "poetic" of the tragic dramatists in the Restoration period. His twelve tragedies (on characters drawn chiefly from classical and Renaissance history) exude figurative language. Tropes flowed from his pen, reaching a torrent of passionate utterance, with the result that his prolific imagery became both his strength and his weakness. The following passage from Act 3 of his *Lucius Junius Brutus* will illustrate his fondness for clusters of imagery:

As in that glass of nature thou shalt view
Thy swoln drown'd eyes with the inverted banks,
The tops of Willows and their blossoms turn'd,
With all the Under Sky ten fathom down,
Wish that the shaddow of the swimming Globe
Were so indeed, that thou migh'st leap at Fate.

All his works are characterized by overcharged emotion and verbal extravagance; furthermore, the hysterical emphasis on passion was rarely balanced by any change of pace or variation of manner. He was fond of spectacle, on-stage tortures, and melodramatic turns. His early plays betray a heavy indebtedness to Elizabethan revenge tragedy and to the bombastic "love and honor" drama of his own time. However, he broke away from these influences to develop his own style, and in *The Rival Queens* he used blank verse and thus abandoned the heroic rhymed couplet before Dryden did.

His own genius showed itself in the depiction of his heroines – Sophonisba, Rosalinda, Statira, Roxana – and in his return to the high road of English tragedy in emphasising the complex character of the protagonist and presenting interior conflict. In *Caesar Borgia*, produced during the anti-Catholic frenzy of 1679, when one would expect only rant and a stereotyped villain, Lee portrays in Borgia (as Allardyce Nicoll says) a struggle "of manliness and vicious influence, of conscience warring against the pernicious atmosphere." Even more dramatic is Alexander in Lee's masterpiece, *The Rival Queens*, a strong protagonist who is torn by internal conflicts and by flaws in his character. The resultant catastrophe is not predetermined but brought on by his own actions. In *Lucius Junius Brutus*, Lee achieved new heights with a drama of ideas, presenting, as James Sutherland says, "a historical tragedy that had a disquieting relevance to contemporary England." Artistically, Brutus seems as fully realised as Addison's Cato but in 1680 no government official stood ready to give the actor £50, as Bolingbroke rewarded Booth; instead, the government banned the play. We ought no longer accept that political verdict as a critical evaluation of the play and should instead recognize the merits of Lee as a tragic dramatist.

In addition, Lee wrote a remarkable "sex" comedy, *The Princess of Cleve*, in the satiric tradition of Wycherley's *The Plain Dealer*, Dryden's *Mr. Limberham*, and Otway's *Friendship in Fashion*. Montague Summers, many years ago, and Robert Hume, in his recent *Development of English Drama*, both show that in the character of Nemours (a comedy of manners "gallant") Lee offers a hostile, even savage depiction of Lord Rochester. Those critics who deny the existence of satire in Restoration drama should read this play.

—Arthur H. Scouten

---

**LILLO, George.** English. Born in Moorfields, London, 4 February 1693. Very little is known about his life: Partner in his father's jewelry business in the City of London; began writing for the theatre c. 1730. *Died 3 September 1739.*

PUBLICATIONS

Collections

*Works.* 2 vols., 1775.

Plays

Silvia; or, The Country Burial (produced 1730). 1730.
The London Merchant; or, The History of George Barnwell (produced 1731). 1731;
   edited by William H. McBurney, 1965.
The Christian Hero (produced 1735). 1735.
Fatal Curiosity (produced 1736; as Guilt Its Own Punishment, produced 1736). 1737;
   edited by William H. McBurney, 1966.
Marina, from the play Pericles by Shakespeare (produced 1738). 1738.
Elmerick; or, Justice Triumphant (produced 1740). 1740.
Britannia and Batavia. 1740.
Arden of Faversham, completed by John Hoadly, from the anonymous play (produced
   1759). 1762.


Reading List: Introduction by Adolphus W. Ward to The London Merchant and Fatal
Curiosity, 1906; Lillo und Siene Bedeutung für die Geschichte des Englischen Dramas by G.
Loccack, 1939; "Notes for a Biography of Lillo" by D. B. Pallette, and "Further Notes" by C.
F. Burgess, in Philological Quarterly, 1940, 1967.

*     *     *

George Lillo is a dramatist who was once immensely popular and influential, but who has
not held the stage for a long time and is now virtually unactable because of the melodramatic
and sentimental qualities of his work. Today his plays are almost unknown except to students
of the eighteenth century, yet in his time he was an artistic innovator, although not the
revolutionary figure in the history of drama he was once thought to be. The view that Lillo
pioneered "bourgeois" tragedy almost single-handed is no longer tenable, but it remains true
that in the play with which his name is always linked, The London Merchant; or, The History
of George Barnwell, he developed a form of domestic tragedy in prose about middle-class life
that is the precursor of the social drama of Ibsen and his successors. Lillo inherited a tradition
of domestic tragedy descending from the Elizabethan theatre and proceeded to modify it in
such a way as to make it conform to the increasingly widespread philosophical and ethical
tenets of sentimentalism and benevolism, while at the same time making it reflect the
concerns of the merchant class. Judging by the almost ecstatic way it was received at the time
of its first production, it is obvious that The London Merchant, like Steele's slightly earlier and
equally popular and influential "sentimental" comedy The Conscious Lovers (1722),
responded to an unspoken demand for a new kind of serious drama, radically different from
the dominant types of comedy and tragedy, still heavily influenced by late seventeenth-
century modes. Subsequently The London Merchant was championed by Continental
intellectuals, being highly praised by Rousseau and Diderot in France and imitated by Lessing
in Germany. Lessing's enthusiasm for Lillo was shared by such prominent members of the
next generation of German writers as Goethe and Schiller, and, particularly through his other
original domestic tragedy, Fatal Curiosity, Lillo exerted a decisive influence on the growth of
German Schicksalstragödie (tragedy of fate) at the end of the eighteenth century. To modern
critics, Lillo's influence seems out of proportion to the instrinsic value of his plays but there is
no denying that he is a dramatist of considerable historical significance.

As has been noted, domestic tragedy was by no means new in the 1730's. There are a
number of Elizabethan and Jacobean examples, including such fine plays as Heywood's A
Woman Killed with Kindness and the anonymous A Yorkshire Tragedy and Arden of
Feversham, and certain late seventeenth- and early eighteenth-century dramatists, notably
Otway, Banks, Southerne, and Rowe, wrote tragedies much more domestic and pathetic than
heroic and classical in conception. Yet these Restoration and Augustan plays do not deal with
everyday English life and could not be called "bourgeois." Whereas prose comedy usually

dealt with contemporary life and ordinary people, poetic tragedy almost invariably adhered to the neoclassical principle that only characters of high birth and social or political eminence, preferably historically or geographically remote ones, could be tragic protagonists. Following the example of Aaron Hill in *The Fatal Extravagance* (1721), ten years before *The London Merchant*, Lillo shattered this doctrine, but whereas Hill's play is a reworking of *A Yorkshire Tragedy*, Lillo's play, which is based on an old ballad and has no dramatic source, is a more conscious attempt to break new ground. The idea of a London apprentice being a tragic hero would have seemed incongruous or even ludicrous to many people at the time, and it is said that some people went to the theatre to sneer, but Lillo won even the sceptics over and his success established that even humble members of society and their private lives were deserving of tragic treatment. Also indicative of his artistic daring is his choice of the medium of comedy, prose; and even though his prose is heightened and sometimes indistinguishable from blank verse it is a decisive step towards greater naturalism in tragic drama and so towards Büchner and Ibsen.

As a tragedy *The London Merchant* is as didactic as a Morality play, contains propaganda on behalf of the merchant class, is incorrigibly sentimental in its treatment of Barnwell's guilt and remorse, and blurs his responsibility for his actions by making him a victim of a power outside himself, the ruthless woman who has led him astray, Millwood. Consequently he is as much a wronged innocent as a culpable human being, even though he is involved in theft and murders his uncle. Many critics have found Lillo's other important play, *Fatal Curiosity*, superior to *The London Merchant* as a domestic tragedy, even though he reverts to blank verse. The provincial setting of *Fatal Curiosity*, the Cornish port of Penryn, makes it more unconventional for a tragedy of its time than the earlier play. As the title suggests, the role of fate is very pronounced, much more so than in *The London Merchant*, and the characters seem to be the helpless playthings and unfortunate victims of fortune. There are certainly no villains. It is out of desperation and necessity and as an alternative to suicide rather than for any evil motive that a destitute, old couple murder an apparent stranger for his wealth, only to discover that he is their long-lost son, a virtuous man of sensibility who has returned in order to help his parents. From the tragic irony of this situation, Lillo extracts a great deal of sentiment. This kind of tragedy of fate was beginning to become popular in the eighteenth century before Lillo, but with this play he did more than any other single dramatist to consolidate it. Discussion of Lillo's interest in domestic tragedy would be incomplete without mentioning his *Arden of Feversham*, staged posthumously in 1759 and obviously based on the Elizabethan play of the same name. The substantial changes Lillo makes in tone and characterization are symptomatic of the impact of sentimentalism on contemporary tragedy, the result being a softening of the tragic intensity of the original. In particular Arden's wife is transformed, so that instead of being the determined and callous prime mover of her husband's murder she is an essentially compassionate woman dominated by her ruthless lover.

Lillo's five other extant dramatic works are of lesser importance (the manuscript of his unpublished comedy, *The Regulators*, was lost in the eighteenth century). His first play, *Silvia*, is a ballad opera in form, but differs from the general run of such works in its moral seriousness and sentimentalism, being about the victory of virtue over vice and the reformation of a libertine. *The Christian Hero* and *Elmerick; or, Justice Triumphant*, both of which have foreign settings, are more conventional tragedies than *The London Merchant* and *Fatal Curiosity*. The first is true to its title in being heroic in conception and idiom, while the second is more deeply tinged with sentiment and pathos. *Marina* is an adaptation of Shakespeare's *Pericles*, while the short masque, *Britannia and Batavia*, is a political allegory. None of these works attracted much attention at the time, and they add almost nothing to his achievement in developing domestic tragedy.

—Peter Lewis

**MACKLIN, Charles.** Irish. Born in Culdaff, Inishowen, in 1699. Educated in a school at Island Bridge, near Dublin. Married 1) Ann Grace in 1739 (died, 1758), one son and one daughter; 2) Elizabeth Jones in 1759 (died, 1781). Lived in London, working in a public house in the Borough district; Badgeman, or Scout, at Trinity College, Dublin, 1713; subsequently joined a strolling company of actors in Bristol; debut as an actor, London, 1725; played with the Drury Lane Company, 1733, the Haymarket Company, 1734, and again with Drury Lane, 1734–48; accidentally killed a fellow actor, tried for murder and acquitted, 1735; taught acting from 1743; appeared in Dublin for Sheridan, 1748–50, and at Covent Garden, London, 1750 until his retirement from the stage, 1753; proprietor of a tavern and coffee house in Covent Garden, 1754–58; returned to the stage, 1759, and continued to act in London, and occasionally in Dublin, until he again retired, 1789. *Died 11 July 1797.*

PUBLICATIONS

Collections

*Four Comedies* (includes *Love A-la-Mode, The True-Born Irishman, The School for Husbands, The Man of the World*), edited by J. O. Bartley. 1968.

Plays

*King Henry VII; or, The Popish Imposter* (produced 1746). 1746.
*A Will and No Will; or, A Bone for the Lawyers*, from a play by J. F. Regnard (produced 1746). Edited by Jean B. Kern, with *The New Play Criticized*, 1967.
*The New Play Criticized; or, The Plague of Envy* (produced 1747). Edited by Jean B. Kern, with *A Will and No Will*, 1967.
*The Club of Fortune-Hunters; or, The Widow Bewitched* (produced 1748).
*The Lover's Melancholy*, from the play by Ford (produced 1748).
*Covent Garden Theatre; or, Pasquin Turned Drawcansir, Censor of Great Britain* (produced 1752). Edited by Jean B. Kern, 1965.
*Love A-la-Mode* (produced 1759). 1784; in *Four Comedies*, 1968.
*The School for Husbands; or, The Married Libertine* (produced 1761). In *Four Comedies*, 1968.
*The True-Born Irishman; or, The Irish Fine Lady* (produced 1762; revised version, as *The Irish Fine Lady*, produced 1767). In *Plays*, 1793; in *Four Comedies*, 1968.
*The Man of the World* (as *The True Born Scotsman*, produced 1764; revised version, as *The Man of the World*, produced 1781). 1785; in *Four Comedies*, 1968.
*The Whim; or, A Christmas Gambol* (produced 1764).
*Plays.* 1793.

Other

*The Case of Charles Macklin, Comedian.* 1743.
*Mr. Macklin's Reply to Mr. Garrick's Answer.* 1743.
*Epistle from Tully in the Shades to Orator M—n in Covent Garden.* 1755.
*An Apology for the Conduct of Mr. Charles Macklin, Comedian.* 1773.
*The Genuine Arguments for a Conspiracy to Deprive Charles Macklin of His Livelihood.* 1774.

*Riot and Conspiracy: The Trial of Thomas Leigh and Others for Conspiring to Ruin in His Profession Charles Macklin.* 1775.

Reading List: *Macklin: An Actor's Life* by William W. Appleton, 1960; "The Comic Plays of Macklin: Dark Satire at Mid-18th Century" by R. R. Findlay, in *Educational Theatre Journal,* 1968.

*       *       *

Charles Macklin was more important to the eighteenth-century English stage as an actor than as a playwright, and his plays frequently adopt the actor's perspective on the world. All ten of them (nine comedies and the ill-starred *Henry VII*) were composed during a busy theatrical career, either as a vehicle for himself or for someone else in the profession, and all are directed towards audiences, not readers. They keep reverting to the nature of the dramatic illusion – whether the stage presents an imitation of our reality, some other reality, or simply unreality – which was also debated by the critics of the time. *A Will and No Will* begins with a "Prologue by the Pit" in which some "members of the audience" onstage discuss the play to come, concluding that they will now see "a Prologue by the Pit." Similarly, at the end of *The New Play Criticized* Heartly asks Lady Critic to write a farce based on the events of the last hour and called *The New Play Criticized*; it will close with his marriage to her daughter. She agrees, and thus Heartly wins his Harriet. Another Harriet, the heroine of *The School for Husbands*, informs Lord Belville that he has been the victim of an elaborate charade by telling him, "We have all been acting a sort of comedy at your expence." More than half of Macklin's comedies play at confusing, at least momentarily, the boundaries commonly supposed to divide life from dramatic art.

This preoccupation is understandable in a man whose consciousness must have been almost wholly histrionic, whose life was the fixed backdrop of Georgian theatre. His acting career spanned sixty-five years, from the days of Cibber and Quin and *The Beggar's Opera*, fifteen years before Garrick's début, to the dawn of melodrama a dozen years after the latter's death. He worked with Fielding at the Haymarket before the Licensing Act, evolved the naturalistic Shylock that made Pope exclaim, "This is the Jew/That Shakespeare drew," tutored Sam Foote in acting, watched Goldsmith and Sheridan come and go, gave some of the earliest lessons in ensemble playing, and opened as the star of his own last comedy when over eighty. On the whole his influence on eighteenth-century theatre rivals Garrick's.

Macklin's forte as a dramatist was a particular kind of verisimilitude: on occasion he commanded the energy to "bounce" an audience into belief in his illusion, as Forster said a novelist should do. He could take a conventional scene (e.g., social climbing in *The True-Born Irishman*, raking and exposure in *The School for Husbands*) and bring it alive through his mastery of colloquial speech and his eye for realistic detail. Had he been able to do this more often we should have heard and thought more of him.

Macklin's best-known full-scale comedy was and is *The Man of the World*, an interesting if flawed prototype of the Victorian problem play; Sir Pertinax Macsycophant, played by Macklin, remains a powerful character. More successful are his short satiric afterpieces, particularly *Love A-la-Mode*, his most popular and lucrative work. The classic testing of Charlotte's four humorous suitors – the fop, the horsey squire, the Scot, and the Teague – gave Macklin an opportunity for writing some of his best dialogue and provided him with a symmetrical structure. The farce as a whole gives an accurate idea of what Macklin could and could not do. It concludes with Sir Callaghan O'Brallaghan remarking that "the whole business is something like the catastrophe of a stage play": another involuted reminder of Macklin's profession.

—R. W. Bevis

**MOORE, Edward.** English.    Born in Abingdon, Berkshire, 22 March 1712. Educated by his uncle, a schoolmaster in Bridgwater, Somerset, and at a school in East Orchard, Dorset. Married Jenny Hamilton in 1749; one son. Apprenticed to a linendraper in London, then worked as a factor in Ireland, then returned to London to set up as a linendraper on his own: turned to literature when the business failed; enjoyed the patronage of Lord Lyttelton: through Lyttelton's influence appointed Editor of *The World* magazine, 1753–56. *Died 1 March 1757.*

PUBLICATIONS

Collections

*Poetical Works*, edited by Thomas Park.    1806.

Plays

*Solomon: A Serenata*, music by William Boyce (produced 1743).    1750.
*The Foundling* (produced 1748).    1748.
*Gil Blas*, from the novel by Le Sage (produced 1751).    1751.
*The Gamester* (produced 1753).    1753.

Verse

*Fables for the Female Sex*.    1744.
*The Trial of Selim the Persian for Divers High Crimes and Misdemeanors*.    1748.
*An Ode to David Garrick*.    1749.

Other

*The World*, with others.    6 vols., 1755–57.
*Poems, Fables, and Plays*.    1756.

Reading List: *The Life and Works of Moore* by John H. Caskey, 1927; Introduction by Charles H. Peake to *The Gamester*, 1948.

\*        \*        \*

It is not hard to see how George Lillo's *George Barnwell; or, The London Merchant* (1731) was one of the greatest hits of the eighteenth-century London stage. The most significant of later eighteenth-century dramatists in the line of Lillo was Edward Moore, best-known as the author of the bourgeois prose tragedy *The Gamester*. The *Poems, Fables, and Plays* show he had wider scope, but it is as a dramatist of domestic dolors that he stands out in John H. Caskey's study and in literary history. He is an important link between Lillo and what came after.

True, he has a secure place in the history of the journalistic essay. After Johnson's *Rambler* and Hawksworth's *Adventurer* came over 200 numbers of *The World* (1753–56) which

Moore edited. He wrote a lot of it himself and attracted contributors such as Chesterfield, Horace Walpole, Soame Jenyns, Richard Owen Cambridge, and Hanbury Williams.

But it was when he went bankrupt as a London linen-draper that Moore came into the theatre and into his own. *Gil Blas* is a lively comedy of disguise based on an episode of Le Sage in which a young lady dresses up as a student in order to capture a man who has caught her eye. Moore adequately handles the quick changes of the young lady back and forth but lacks the verbal lightness for really effective quick exchanges of dialogue. The borrowed plot remains the redeeming feature.

*The Foundling* was more in Moore's style, a sentimental and moral excursion along the lines that Cibber had more or less invented and Steele had made more or less popular, an earnest endeavor such as Moore's friend Fielding has his Parson Adams damn with feinting praise like this: "there are some things almost solemn enough for a sermon." The remark may underline for us how far comedy had strayed at that period from corrective laughter. If comedy was full of fine feeling and nearly devoid of fun, just imagine the domestic tragedy between, say, *The London Merchant* and Kelly's *False Delicacy*. *The Foundling* was nominally a comedy but is hardly a laugh riot. I find the work with which Moore started to make money as a writer, *Fables for the Female Sex*, funnier. The play is well constructed, however.

Then when Garrick (who played in it) gave Moore a hand with *The Gamester*, Moore had a first-rate piece of its kind. If you have tears, prepare to shed them now as we note the sad story of Beverley, a victim (like Barnwell) of evil in the vile form of Stukeley (who owes something to Lillo's Millwood, something to Shakespeare's Iago, and something to Fielding's Jonathan Wild). Beverley is sunk in a mire of gambling debts. Under the mercantile ethic (presented in numerous middle-class plays as well as in novels from Defoe and others throughout the century) squandering money was the foulest of crimes. In a comedy, by some stratagem finances as well as love affairs all come right in the end. In this tragedy, Beverley poisons himself in despair just before it transpires that he was to inherit the estate of his rich uncle! The distraught Mrs. Beverley wrings every drop of sentiment out of her husband's fate, though the play is not a "she-tragedy" of the Otway or Rowe variety. It is rather in the Elizabethan tradition of domestic melodrama and a milestone in the "road to ruin" genre which began to concentrate more and more not on the gambler himself but, as in temperance dramas, on the dire effects upon guiltless wives and suffering children.

The weakness in the genre is that the gambler is generally either a villain (in which case he attracts no sympathy) or a sap (like Barnwell or Beverley). It is hard to bring naturalism to the hysteria and histrionics. Moore's dialogue is more "natural" than Lillo's, but what Goldsmith would have called "natural" (as when he spoke of Garrick's "simple, natural, affecting" acting) may look pretty stilted and posturing to us.

Diderot adapted *The Gamester* as a *drame bourgeois* and Thomas Holcroft echoed some aspects of Moore in *The Road to Ruin* (1792). Moore's play has relevance to all the sentimental plays of the latter part of the eighteenth century and all the melodramatic ones of the first half of the nineteenth century; in its confusion of tragic hero and hapless victim, of sentiment and seriousness, of tragedy and melodrama, it is related to such works as Arthur Miller's *Death of a Salesman*. *The Gamester* is a masterpiece of the second-rate and as such of first-rate importance in the history of the theatre.

—Leonard R. N. Ashley

---

**MORTON, Thomas.** English. Born in Durham c. 1764. Educated at Soho Square School, London; entered Lincoln's Inn, 1784, but was not subsequently admitted to the bar. Married; one daughter and two sons, including the playwright John Maddison Morton. Full-time playwright from 1792. Senior Member of Lord's, London; Honorary Member, Garrick Club, 1837. *Died 28 March 1838.*

PUBLICATIONS

Plays

*Columbus; or, A World Discovered* (produced 1792). 1792.

*The Children in the Wood*, music by Samuel Arnold (produced 1793). 1794.

*Zorinski*, music by Samuel Arnold (produced 1795). 1795.

*The Way to Get Married* (produced 1796). 1796.

*A Cure for the Heart-Ache* (produced 1797). 1797.

*Secrets Worth Knowing* (produced 1798). 1798.

*Speed the Plough* (produced 1800). 1800; edited by Allardyce Nicoll in *Lesser English Comedies of the Eighteenth Century*, 1931.

*The Blind Girl; or, A Receipt for Beauty*, music by Joseph Massinghi and William Reeve (produced 1801). Songs published 1801.

*Beggar My Neighbour; or, A Rogue's a Fool*, from a play by A. W. Iffland (produced 1802; as *How to Tease and How to Please*, produced 1810).

*The School of Reform; or, How to Rule a Husband* (produced 1805). 1805.

*Town and Country* (produced 1807). 1807.

*The Knight of Snowdoun*, music by Henry Bishop, from the poem "The Lady of the Lake" by Scott (produced 1811). 1811.

*Education* (produced 1813). 1813.

*The Slave*, music by Henry Bishop (produced 1816). 1816.

*Methinks I See My Father; or, Who's My Father?* (produced 1818). 1850(?).

*A Roland for an Oliver*, from a play by Scribe (produced 1819). 1819.

*Henri Quatre; or, Paris in the Olden Time*, music by Henry Bishop (produced 1820). 1820.

*A School for Grown Children* (produced 1827). 1827.

*The Invincibles*, music by A. Lee (produced 1828). 1829.

*The Sublime and Beautiful* (produced 1828).

*Peter the Great; or, The Battle of Pultawa*, with James Kenney, music by Tom Cooke and William Carnaby, from a play by Frédéric du Petit-Mère (produced 1829).

*Separation and Reparation* (produced 1830).

*The King's Fireside* (produced 1830).

*The Writing on the Wall!*, with J. M. Morton (produced 1852). N.d.

\*   \*   \*

Thomas Morton's first five-act comedy, *The Way to Get Married*, gave good acting parts to Lewis, Quick, Munden, and Fawcett. It also established his method, which is to embed a pathetic tale of poverty and remorse amid comic episodes and eccentric characters. Scenes of convulsive anguish alternate with amusing encounters and adventures whose general intention is to commend generosity and expose the mercenary motives of a heartless society. Morton was, in effect, writing melodrama before the word had reached the English theatre. He had, generally, the tact to give his comedians more stage time than his "heavies," and to allow one of his comic men to make the crucial discovery that makes all well. *Secrets Worth Knowing* is an exact example of the style. The comedy survives well, but the suffering resists contemporary staging. The same is true of Morton's best play, *Speed the Plough*, in which the real life belongs to the characters least involved in the main plot. Sir Philip Blandford's remorse over a dead wife, lost child, and murdered brother is tediously related in embarrassingly pompous prose. The child (not lost), the brother (not murdered), and the daughter also speak in grandiose archaisms. By extraordinary contrast, the uxorious Sir Abel Handy, his well-intentioned son, his wife, Farmer and Mrs. Ashfield, and their daughter are all finely observed and provided with sprightly dialogue. It is Mrs. Ashfield's obsessive concern with what Mrs. Grundy (who never appears) may say that has provided Morton's best known monument. *The School of Reform* is an attempt to repeat the success of *Speed the Plough*, but the influence of the German dramatists, particularly of Kotzebue's guilt-laden stories of sexual sin, swamps most of Morton's own talent. The character of Robert Tyke, and the final sensation scene in a Gothic chapel, underline the close relations between contemporary comedy and melodrama. *A Cure for the Heart-Ache* is the only one of Morton's comedies to suit the description, though even that play is not without pathetic attitudinising.

—Peter Thomson

---

**MURPHY, Arthur.** Irish. Born in Clomquin, Roscommon, 27 December 1727; lived with his family in Dublin, 1729–35, and in London from 1735. Studied at the English College in St. Omer, France, 1738–44. Clerk to a merchant in Cork, 1747–49; worked in the City banking house of Ironside and Belchier, London, 1749–51; publisher of, and leading contributor to, *Gray's Inn Journal*, 1752–54; appeared as an actor at Covent Garden and Drury Lane, 1754–55, and began writing for the stage, 1756; admitted to Lincoln's Inn, London, 1757, was subsequently called to the bar, and practised in London; also edited the weekly papers, *The Test* and *The Auditor*; retired from the law and the theatre, 1788; appointed a commissioner of bankrupts and granted a pension by George III, 1803. *Died 18 June 1805.*

PUBLICATIONS

Collections

*The Way to Keep Him and Five Other Plays* (includes *The Apprentice, The Upholsterer, The Old Maid, Three Weeks after Marriage, Know Your Own Mind*), edited by John P. Emery. 1956.

Plays

*The Apprentice* (produced 1756). 1756; in *The Way to Keep Him and Five Other Plays*, 1956.
*The Englishman from Paris* (produced 1756).
*The Upholsterer; or, What News?* (produced 1758). 1758; edited by R. W. Bevis, in *Eighteenth Century Drama: Afterpieces*, 1970.
*The Orphan of China*, from a play by Voltaire (produced 1759). 1759.
*The Tears and Triumphs of Parnassus*, with Robert Lloyd, music by John Stanley (produced 1760).
*The Way to Keep Him*, from a play by Moissy (produced 1760). 1760; revised version (produced 1761), 1761; in *The Way to Keep Him and Five Other Plays*, 1956; 1760 version edited by R. W. Bevis, in *Eighteenth Century Drama: Afterpieces*, 1970.

*The Desert Island*, from a play by Metastasio (produced 1760).   1760.
*All in the Wrong* (produced 1761).   1761.
*The Old Maid*, from a play by Fagan (produced 1761).   1761.
*The Citizen*, from a play by Destouches (produced 1761).   1763.
*No One's Enemy But His Own*, from a play by Voltaire (produced 1764).   1764.
*What We Must All Come To* (produced 1764).   1764; as *Three Weeks after Marriage* (produced 1776), 1776; in *The Way to Keep Him and Five Other Plays*, 1956.
*The Choice* (produced 1765).   In *Works*, 1786.
*The School for Guardians*, from a play by Molière (produced 1767).   1767.
*Zenobia* (produced 1768).   1768.
*The Grecian Daughter* (produced 1772).   1772.
*Alzuma* (produced 1773).   1773.
*News from Parnassus* (produced 1776).   In *Works*, 1786.
*Know Your Own Mind*, from a play by Destouches (produced 1777).   1778; in *The Way to Keep Him and Five Other Plays*, 1956.
*The Rival Sisters* (produced 1793).   In *Works*, 1786.
*Arminius*.   1798.
*Hamlet, with Alterations*, from the play by Shakespeare, in *Life of Murphy* by J. Foot. 1811; edited by Martin Lehnert, in *Shakespeare Jahrbuch 102*, 1966.

Verse

*A Poetical Epistle to Samuel Johnson.*   1760.
*An Ode to the Naiads of Fleet Ditch.*   1761.
*The Examiner: A Satire.*   1761.
*Seventeen Hundred and Ninety-One: A Poem in Imitation of the Thirteenth Satire of Juvenal.*   1791.
*The Bees: A Poem from the Fourteenth Book of Vaniere's Praedium Rusticum.*   1799.
*The Game of Chess*, from a poem by Vida.   1876.

Other

*The Gray's Inn Journal.*   2 vols., 1756.
*A Letter to Voltaire on The Desert Island.*   1760.
*Works.*   7 vols., 1786.
*An Essay on the Life and Genius of Samuel Johnson.*   1792.
*The Life of David Garrick.*   2 vols., 1801.
*New Essays*, edited by Arthur Sherbo.   1963.

Editor, *Works*, by Fielding.   4 vols., 1762.

Translator, *The Works of Tacitus.*   4 vols., 1793.
Translator, *The Works of Sallust.*   1807.

Reading List: *Murphy: An Eminent English Dramatist of the Eighteenth Century* by John P. Emery, 1946; *The Dramatic Career of Murphy* by Howard Hunter Dunbar, 1946; Introduction by Simon Trefman to *The Englishman from Paris*, 1969.

\*      \*      \*

A man of broad interests and a prolific writer, Arthur Murphy was a journalist, biographer, editor, actor, translator of the classics, lawyer, political writer, and one of the most successful playwrights of the third quarter of the eighteenth century. Of particular interest among Murphy's various non-dramatic writings are his *Gray's Inn Journal* and biographies of Garrick, Fielding, and Johnson. These works contain much perceptive practical criticism, Murphy's generally traditional literary theories, and a great deal of information about the theater and literary life of his age.

About twenty of Murphy's plays were performed during the eighteenth century. These range from short farces and satires used as afterpieces to full-length tragedies and comedies. Although at least minimally successful in all the dramatic genres he attempted, Murphy's greatest skill is evident in his comedies and farces. One of the best of these is *The Way to Keep Him*, which was first performed as a three-act afterpiece and was a miniature comedy, not a farce. After Murphy rewrote it in five acts, the resulting full-fledged comedy of manners remained popular for a century. The play, which deals with various modes of marital behavior, contains some sentimental elements, but generally shares the same spirit as the comedies of Congreve and Sheridan. *All in the Wrong*, *The School for Guardians*, and *Know Your Own Mind* also display Murphy's talent for writing comedies of manners.

Murphy's farces are among the best in an age that is noted for good farces. Whether focusing on satire or outlandish situations, his farces are usually fast-paced and his characters, often "humours" types, well-drawn. *The Apprentice* and *The Upholsterer* satirize stage-struck apprentices and tradesmen who are excessively interested in politics, respectively. The latter contains a character, Mrs. Termagant, who may have been a source for Sheridan's Mrs. Malaprop. Other farces worthy of mention are *The Old Maid*, *No One's Enemy But His Own*, and *Three Weeks after Marriage*. The ingenious situational humor and riotous quarrel scenes make the latter an especially lively theatrical piece.

—James S. Malek

---

**O'KEEFFE, John.** Irish. Born in Dublin, 24 June 1747. Educated at a Jesuit school in Saul's Court, Dublin; afterwards studied art in the Dublin School of Design. Married; one daughter and two sons. Originally an actor: member of Henry Mossop's stock company, Dublin, 1762–74; wrote for the stage from 1767; settled in London, c. 1780, and thereafter wrote comic pieces for the Haymarket and Covent Garden theatres; blind from the mid-1780's; received an annuity from Covent Garden, 1803, and a royal pension, 1820. *Died 4 February 1833.*

PUBLICATIONS

Plays

> *The She Gallant; or, Square-Toes Outwitted* (produced 1767). 1767; revised version, as *The Positive Man*, music by Samuel Arnold and Michael Arne (produced 1782), in *Dramatic Works*, 1798.
> *Colin's Welcome* (produced 1770).
> *Tony Lumpkin in Town* (produced 1774). 1780.

*The Poor Soldier* (as *The Shamrock, or, St. Patrick's Day,* produced 1777; revised version, as *The Poor Soldier,* music by William Shield, produced 1783). 1785.

*The Son-in-Law,* music by Samuel Arnold (produced 1779). 1783.

*The Dead Alive,* music by Samuel Arnold (produced 1781). 1783.

*The Agreeable Surprise,* music by Samuel Arnold (produced 1781). 1784.

*The Banditti; or, Love's Labyrinth,* music by Samuel Arnold (produced 1781). Songs published 1781; revised version, as *The Castle of Andalusia* (produced 1782), 1783; revised version (produced 1788).

*Harlequin Teague; or, The Giant's Causeway,* music by Samuel Arnold (produced 1782). Songs published 1782.

*Lord Mayor's Day; or, A Flight from Lapland,* music by William Shield (produced 1782). Songs published 1782.

*The Maid the Mistress,* from a play by G. A. Federico (produced 1783). Songs published 1783.

*The Young Quaker* (produced 1783). 1784.

*The Birthday; or, The Prince of Arragon,* music by Samuel Arnold, from a play by Saint-Foix (produced 1783). 1783.

*Gretna Green* (lyrics only), play by Charles Stuart, music by Samuel Arnold (produced 1783). 1791.

*Friar Bacon; or, Harlequin's Adventures in Lilliput, Brobdignag etc.* (lyrics only), play by Charles Bonner, music by William Shield (produced 1783; as *Harlequin Rambler,* produced 1784). Songs published 1784.

*Peeping Tom of Coventry,* music by Samuel Arnold (produced 1784). 1786.

*Fontainbleau; or, Our Way in France,* music by William Shield (produced 1784). 1785.

*The Blacksmith of Antwerp* (produced 1785). In *Dramatic Works,* 1798.

*A Beggar on Horseback,* music by Samuel Arnold (produced 1785). In *Dramatic Works,* 1798.

*Omai; or, A Trip round the World,* music by William Shield (produced 1785). Songs published 1785.

*Love in a Camp; or, Patrick in Prussia,* music by William Shield (produced 1786). 1786.

*The Siege of Curzola,* music by Samuel Arnold (produced 1786). Songs published 1786.

*The Man Milliner* (produced 1787). In *Dramatic Works,* 1798.

*Love and War,* from the play *The Campaign* by Robert Jephson (produced 1787).

*The Farmer,* music by William Shield (produced 1787). 1788.

*Tantara-Rara, Rogues All,* from a play by Dumaniant (produced 1788). In *Dramatic Works,* 1798.

*The Prisoner at Large* (produced 1788). 1788.

*The Highland Reel,* music by William Shield (produced 1788). 1789.

*Aladdin; or, The Wonderful Lamp,* music by William Shield (produced 1788). Songs published 1788.

*The Lie of the Day* (as *The Toy,* produced 1789; revised version, as *The Lie of the Day,* produced 1796). In *Dramatic Works,* 1798.

*The Faro Table,* from the play *The Gamester* by Mrs. Centlivre (produced 1789).

*The Little Hunch-Back; or, A Frolic in Bagdad* (produced 1789). 1789.

*The Czar Peter,* music by William Shield (as *The Czar,* produced 1790; as *The Fugitive,* produced 1790). In *Dramatic Works,* 1798.

*The Basket-Maker,* music by Samuel Arnold (produced 1790). In *Dramatic Works,* 1798.

*Modern Antiques; or, The Merry Mourners* (produced 1791). 1792.

*Wild Oats; or, The Strolling Gentleman* (produced 1791). 1791; edited by Clifford Williams, 1977.

*Tony Lumpkin's Ramble to Town* (produced 1792).
*Sprigs of Laurel,* music by William Shield (produced 1793).    1793; revised version, as
    *The Rival Soldiers* (produced 1797).
*The London Hermit; or, Rambles in Dorsetshire* (produced 1793).    1793.
*The World in a Village* (produced 1793).    1793.
*Life's Vagaries* (produced 1795).    1795.
*The Irish Mimic; or, Blunders at Brighton,* music by William Shield (produced
    1795).    1795.
*Merry Sherwood; or, Harlequin Forester* (lyrics only), play by Mark Lonsdale and
    William Pearce, music by William Reeve (produced 1795).    Songs published 1795.
*The Wicklow Gold Mines; or, The Lad of the Hills,* music by William Shield (produced
    1796).    1814; revised version, as *The Wicklow Mountains* (produced 1796), 1797.
*The Doldrum; or, 1803* (produced 1796).    In *Dramatic Works,* 1798.
*Alfred; or, The Magic Banner* (produced 1796).    1796.
*Olympus in an Uproar; or, The Descent of the Deities,* from the play *The Golden Pippin*
    by Kane O'Hara (produced 1796).
*Britain's Brave Tars; or, All for St. Paul's,* music by Thomas Attwood (produced 1797).
*She's Eloped* (produced 1798).
*The Eleventh of June; or, The Daggerwoods at Dunstable* (produced 1798).
*A Nosegay of Weeds; or, Old Servants in New Places* (produced 1798).
*Dramatic Works.*    4 vols., 1798.

Verse

*Oatlands; or, The Transfer of the Laurel.*    1795.
*A Father's Legacy to His Daughter, Being the Poetical Works,* edited by Adelaide
    O'Keeffe.    1834.

Other

*Recollections of the Life of O'Keeffe, Written by Himself.*    2 vols., 1826.

\*       \*       \*

John O'Keeffe wrote for a living, and was the slave of a public about which he must
sometimes have grumbled but which he hated to upset. Between 1778, when the elder
Colman bought for the Haymarket his opportunistic afterpiece *Tony Lumpkin in Town,* and
1800, when Thomas Harris awarded him a benefit at Covent Garden, O'Keeffe was a
provider of theatrical pieces for those two theatres. Most of these pieces depend as much on
song as on dialogue. Of the some 60 he admits to in his *Recollections,* over 20 are called
"operas," a way of assuring contemporary audiences that the dialogue would be frequently
interrupted by songs. In the three acts of *The Castle of Andalusia* there are over 20 such
interruptions. The music for this popular piece was arranged by Dr. Arnold, but borrowed
from Italy, Ireland, and the London streets. The plot calls for a noble bandit, a resourceful
rogue, two pairs of lovers, an ageing and covetous widow, and the audience's ready
acceptance of the convention of gullibility without which plays of mistaken identity will
crumble about their ears. In *Fontainbleau* there are fewer songs and a greater dependence on
bright dialogue and quirky characters like Colonel Epaulette, the anglophile Frenchman who
makes his first entrance singing "Rule Britannia, Britannia rule de vay." The Jonsonian
"humour" is close to journey's end in mere risible eccentricity, although there is comic
resource and energy in O'Keeffe's handling of a slender story. He was bound by convention
to attempt the more exacting five-act comedy form. *The Young Quaker* was moderately

successful at the small Haymarket, and *The Toy*, later reduced to three acts as *The Lie of the Day*, was an effective vehicle for William Lewis, Quick, and Aickin.

But it was *Wild Oats* that made and has preserved O'Keeffe's reputation as a writer of comedy. The play depends on an alias, a carefully contrived mistaken identity, a sequence of coincidences, and a lost baby miraculously rediscovered in the person of the leading character, a strolling player conditionally named Rover. Plot and characters are not original, but if not of invention, there is a sufficient freshness of deployment to explain the success of the 1976 revival by the Royal Shakespeare Company. Rover, who has a dramatic quotation for every emergency, was created by Lewis and has proved the play's main attraction in the theatre. In a reading, the hostility towards Quaker puritanism and a veiled egalitarianism are quite as striking. O'Keeffe was proud to boast of Sheridan's calling him "the first that turned the public taste from the dullness of sentiment ... towards the sprightly channel of comic humour." He was *not* the first, but *Wild Oats* is a substantial alternative to the sentimental plays that surrounded it. Of the three other five-act comedies performed in his lifetime, *She's Eloped* survived only one night while *The World in a Village* and *Life's Vagaries* were moderately successful.

—Peter Thomson

---

**ORRERY, Earl of.** See **BOYLE, Roger.**

---

**OTWAY, Thomas.** English. Born in Trotten, Sussex, 3 March 1652. Educated at Winchester College, Hampshire, 1668; Christ Church, Oxford, 1669–71, left without taking a degree. Served in the Duke of Monmouth's Regiment in the Netherlands, 1678–79. Settled in London, 1671, and worked temporarily as an actor; wrote for the Duke's Company at the Dorset Garden Theatre, London, from 1675. *Died 14 April 1685.*

PUBLICATIONS

Collections

*The Works,* edited by J. C. Ghosh. 2 vols., 1932.

Plays

*Alcibiades* (produced 1675). 1675.
*Don Carlos, Prince of Spain* (produced 1676). 1676.

*Titus and Berenice*, from a play by Racine (produced 1676).    1677.
*The Cheats of Scapin*, from a play by Molière (produced 1676).    In *Titus and Berenice*, 1677.
*Friendship in Fashion* (produced 1678).    1678.
*The History and Fall of Caius Marius* (produced 1679).    1680.
*The Orphan; or, The Unhappy Marriage* (produced 1680).    1680; edited by Aline M. Taylor, 1976.
*The Soldier's Fortune* (produced 1680).    1681.
*Venice Preserved; or, A Plot Discovered* (produced 1682).    1682; edited by Malcolm Kelsall, 1969.
*The Atheist; or, The Second Part of the Soldier's Fortune* (produced 1683).    1684.

Verse

*The Poet's Complaint of His Muse; or, A Satire Against Libels*.    1680.
*Windsor Castle in a Monument to Our Late Sovereign Charles II*.    1685.

Other

*Familiar Letters* (by Rochester, Otway, and Katherine Philips), edited by Tom Brown and Charles Gildon.    2 vols., 1697.

Translator, *The History of the Triumvirates*, by Samuel de Broe.    1686.

Reading List: *Otway and Lee* by Roswell G. Ham, 1931; *Next to Shakespeare* by Aline M. Taylor, 1950; *Gestalt und Funktion der Bilder im Otway und Lee* by Gisela Fried, 1965; *Die Künstlerische Entwicklung in der Tragödien Otways* by Helmut Klinger, 1971.

\*       \*       \*

In the eight years between 1675 and 1683 Thomas Otway wrote and had produced at Dorset Garden Theatre ten plays. Two of his six tragedies are of lasting quality; the other four are of varying merit. The four comedies are generally regarded as having little to recommend them, though a farce entitled *The Cheats of Scapin* held the stage for many years. The first two plays, *Alcibiades* and *Don Carlos*, belong to the prevailing genre of Heroic Tragedy, being written in heroic couplets of elevated rhetoric to be spoken by supremely noble characters, and emphasizing the themes of love, honour, and valour. Yet even in these Otway broke out of the stereotype, especially in the latter play, to create scenes of unaffected sincerity, tenderness, and simplicity. The later tragedies are derived, as was becoming the fashion by 1677, more directly in form and substance from Elizabethan and Jacobean antecedents. His comedies likewise follow, though with less success, Elizabethan and Jacobean structure and variety – brought up to date with fashionable cynicism, vulgarity, and attempts at Restoration wit.

For his direct source Otway went to Plutarch (*Alcibiades*), Racine (*Titus and Berenice*), Molière (*The Cheats of Scapin*), Roger Boyle (*The Orphan*), Shakespeare (*Don Carlos* and *Caius Marius*) and Saint Réal (*Don Carlos*). Just as importantly, he drew in his bitter comedies upon the cynical tone and wit of Wycherley, and upon Shakespeare for the same qualities in all his plays, as well as for dramatic situation, structure, and poetry. Out of his own poverty, disappointment in patronage, unhappy army experience, and hopeless love for Mrs. Barry came also much of his fatalism, cynicism, and despair, tones which fit well the popular Hobbesism of the time. His striking this popular mood of the theatre-goers – the nobles, courtiers, and wits – doubtless accounted for his considerable success in his own day. Furthermore, the slightly veiled parallels and references in his plays (in the comedies and in *Caius Marius* and *Venice Preserved*) to current political intrigues, especially the popish plot and attacks upon the Whigs and the Earl of Shaftesbury, brought patrons to Dorset Garden. But his temperament and his attraction to Shakespeare's special brand of satire perhaps account best for Otway's more lasting qualities.

And his success upon the tragic stage has been considerable. For his two powerful tragedies he has been called "Next to Shakespeare," the title of Aline Taylor's full account of the remarkable stage success of *Venice Preserved* and *The Orphan*. Contributing greatly to this success have been the superb actors who have played the chief roles. But other lasting qualities have contributed to their survival and retained a place for them and the rest of Otway's plays in the history of dramatic literature. Otway became an excellent dramatic craftsman, and he also had something important, though quite unflattering, to say about the human condition.

Otway's exposition usually follows an immediate plunge into the midst of the action, such as the opening quarrel of *Venice Preserved*, which creates effective suspense. The suspense is intensified through the complication, and the direct, swift action brings on the powerful climax. The result is a shattering recognition for the principals, especially in the tragedies, which is followed by an unrelieved dénouement of defeat and despair in the tragedies and only cynicism in the comedies. The movement in the tragedies is often, like that of Greek tragedy, direct and inevitable. In *The Orphan* onlooker and reader alike are held horrified in their anxiety: surely Castalio will tell Polydore that he is married to Monimia; surely someone will light a taper! But the light comes too late; the recognition is too great for the principals to bear, as is also true in *Venice Preserved*, *Don Carlos*, and *Caius Marius*. Such inability reflects the basic fault in Otway's main characters. His dramas rise from the weaknesses of his characters: they are strong in emotion, but weak in judgment, more given to blaming fate than recognizing their own crucial errors – which lead to self-destruction.

This same quality of irresponsibility gave rise to a sort of perverse wit, bitter and sardonic, in both his comedies and tragedies. Inherited from Shakespeare and Marston in large part, it is perhaps best exemplified in *Venice Preserved*. Pierre makes his nervous midnight entrance upon the Rialto for his assignation with Jaffeir. Like Bernardo in *Hamlet*, he improperly challenges the one who is already on the scene: "Speak, who goes there?" He gets the reply: "A dog, that comes to howl/At yonder moon: What's he that asks the Question?" Pierre answers "A Friend to Dogs, for they are honest creatures." (In *Julius Caesar* Brutus reproves Cassius with "I'd rather be a dog and bay the moon/Than such a Roman.") The following speeches revile priesthood and condemn prayer and religion.

This same sort of cynicism in Otway's plays gives rise to numerous oaths, curses, and orations, all of which make for intense dramatic effect. Pierre's notable speech before the Senate asks in four ironic rhetorical questions whether the chains that bind him are "the wreaths of triumph ye bestow," for his service to the state. Jaffeir's solemn oath to remain faithful to the conspiracy becomes ironic as he, for love of Belvidera, fails to keep the oath and then denounces his own failure before the Senate. He curses Old Priuli, as might a primitive Irish satirist: "Kind Heav'n! let heavy Curses/Gall his old Age; Cramps, Aches rack his Bones...." Belvidera calls upon heaven to pour down curses with vengeance, despair, danger, etc. upon her; and Jaffeir in a final curse, such as Polydore's in *The Orphan*, asks that a "Final destruction seize the world...." And this is just what happens to his world as he and Belvidera commit suicide. All is left in ruins. Though one may argue that underlying *Venice Preserved* is the affirmation of the integrity of the family (as one may argue for the same in *Coriolanus*), such integrity does not prevail at the end of the play – only the corrupt Senate prevails. The very title is ironic: Venice preserved indeed!

Just such lack of affirmation, just such lack of hope characterize Otway's plays. Fortune, Chance, Fate control – not men or benevolent gods. Even the earlier *Alcibiades*, *Don Carlos*, and *Caius Marius* lack a just settling of accounts; the comedies, *The Soldier's Fortune* and *The Atheist*, are dissertations upon Fortune and Chance.

The ritualistic use of formal curses, prayers, oaths, and set speeches make Otway's plays dramatically effective. But the sardonic and cynical quality be gives them belong rather to satire than pure comedy or tragedy. As a part of rhetoric, style, and invention this quality reverses the normal processes of expression and appeals both to emotion and intellect. It is inherently dramatic, and Otway uses it with great effect. Yet it cannot rise to affirmation. The conclusions of his plots bring no sense of order or justice having been reasserted. Rather, chaos prevails, and an effective catharsis does not take place. The audience are left to face a meaningless, unintelligible world, anticipating the school of the absurd of the mid-twentieth century.

Otway's dozen poems outside the plays and his half-dozen love letters are useful chiefly in explaining the partisanship, political and historical allusions, and tone of the plays. The love letters reveal in effective, if sometimes maudlin, prose the poet's hopeless passion for Mrs. Barry; hence the character of his tragic heroines. Of the poems, *The Poet's Complaint of His Muse* and *Windsor Castle* seem most significant. The former is autobiographical, consisting of twenty-one strophes shot through with allusions to contemporary events and political affairs. It ends with a tribute to James, Duke of York, as he takes precautionary leave of England because of the Popish Plot. The latter is an extensive panegyric upon the ascension of James II, who "By mighty deeds has earnrown he wears." Both indicate directly the poet's scornful opposition to the Whigs and his sympathy and admiration for the Royalists — attitudes revealed implicitly in his plays.

—Thomas B. Stroup

---

**RAVENSCROFT, Edward.** English. Born in England c. 1650. Very little is known about his life: descended from an ancient Flintshire family; member of the Middle Temple, London, 1671; career as a playwright extended over a quarter century, but he is thought to have died comparatively young: nothing is recorded about him after 1697.

PUBLICATIONS

Plays

> *The Citizen Turned Gentleman*, from a play by Molière (produced 1672).   1672; as *Mamamouchi*, 1675.
> *The Careless Lovers* (produced 1673).   1673.
> *The Wrangling Lovers; or, The Invisible Mistress* (produced 1676).   1677.
> *Scaramouche a Philosopher, Harlequin a School-Boy, Bravo, Merchant and Magician* (produced 1677).   1677.
> *The English Lawyer*, from a Latin play by George Ruggle (produced 1677).   1678.
> *King Edgar and Alfreda* (produced 1677).   1677.
> *The London Cuckolds* (produced 1681).   1682; edited by A. Norman Jeffares, in *Restoration Comedy*, 1974.
> *Dame Dobson; or, The Cunning Woman*, from a play by Thomas Corneille (produced 1683).   1684.

*Titus Andronicus; or, The Rape of Lavinia*, from the play by Shakespeare (produced 1686). 1687.

*The Canterbury Guests; or, A Bargain Broken* (produced 1694). 1695.

*The Anatomist; or, The Sham Doctor* (produced 1696). 1697; edited by Leo Hughes and Arthur H. Scouten, in *Ten English Farces*, 1948.

*The Italian Husband* (produced 1697). 1698.

\*     \*     \*

In the prologue to his *Assignation* Dryden jeered at his rival Edward Ravenscroft for pleasing the crowd but being condemned by the critics for his very first play, *The Citizen Turn'd Gentleman*. The Laureate's judgment proved prophetic. In an age which insisted on interpreting Horace as requiring *edification*, Ravenscroft found his success in *entertainment*.

His early comedies, all following a common Restoration pattern of combining scenes from as many as three plays by Molière, were generally successful. His serious attempts, a play borrowed from early English history, *King Edgar and Alfreda*, an adaptation of Shakespeare's *Titus Andronicus*, and an equally macabre borrowing from the Italian called *The Italian Husband*, won no lasting acclaim. *Scaramouche*, borrowed from both Molière and his *commedia dell'arte* neighbors, anticipates in many ways the vastly popular pantomimes of the next century and provides something of a pattern for his two most successful pieces: *The London Cuckolds*, which lasted 102 years but eventually proved too bawdy for an increasingly squeamish age, and *The Anatomist*, an even livelier but less risqué piece which proved more fortunate in its long theatrical history. *The London Cuckolds* borrows only its theme, the absurdity of attempting by contrivance to avoid even the risk of cuckoldry, from *The School for Wives*, but Ravenscroft multiplies Molière's Arnolphe by three, adds several farce turns wholly unconnected with the French play, and succeeds in being shocking and amusing at one and the same time. Borrowed from Hauteroche but much improved by some additional farce turns of his own, *The Anatomist* was turned into a one-act afterpiece at Goodman's Fields just a few months before David Garrick began his illustrious career at that theatre. *The Anatomist* was a favorite of Garrick's. He repeatedly attached it to his own pieces or to his own performances throughout his career. Beyond Garrick's time it waned somewhat in popularity but lasted until the mid-nineteenth century, well beyond the term of a hundred years which, according to Dr. Johnson's dictum, is "commonly fixed as the test of literary merit." In Ravenscroft's case perhaps *theatrical* merit would be the more appropriate term.

—Leo Hughes

**ROWE, Nicholas.** English. Born in Little Barford, Bedfordshire, baptized 30 June 1674. Educated at Westminster School, London (King's Scholar); entered the Middle Temple, London, 1691. Married Antonia Parons in 1698. Inherited the family estate, 1692, and gave up the law for playwriting; also held various official appointments: Under-Secretary to the Duke of Queensbury, Secretary of State for Scotland, 1709–11. First modern editor of Shakespeare, 1709. Poet Laureate, 1715 until his death. *Died 6 December 1718.*

PUBLICATIONS

Collections

    *Plays* edited by Anne D. Devenish.   2 vols., 1747.
    *Works*.   2 vols., 1764.
    *Three Plays* (includes *Tamerlane, The Fair Penitent, Jane Shore*), edited by James R.
        Sutherland.   1929.

Plays

    *The Ambitious Step-Mother* (produced 1700).   1701.
    *Tamerlane* (produced 1701).   1701; edited by Landon C. Burns, 1966.
    *The Fair Penitent*, from the play *The Fatal Dowry* by Massinger and Nathan Field
        (produced 1703).   1703; edited by Malcolm Goldstein, 1969.
    *The Biter* (produced 1704).   1705.
    *Ulysses* (produced 1705).   1706.
    *The Royal Convert* (produced 1707).   1708; as *Ethelinda* (produced 1776).
    *The Tragedy of Jane Shore* (produced 1714).   1714; edited by Harry William Pedicord,
        1974.
    *Tragedies*.   2 vols., 1714.
    *Lady Jane Gray* (produced 1715).   1715.

Verse

    *A Poem upon the Late Glorious Successes of Her Majesty's Arms*.   1707.
    *Poems on Several Occasions*.   1714.
    *Poetical Works*.   1715.
    *Ode for the New Year 1716*.   1716.
    *Ode for the Year 1717.*   1717.
    *Ode to the Thames for the Year 1719*.   1719.

Other

    Editor, with J. Tonson, *Poetical Miscellanies 5–6*, by Dryden.   2 vols., 1704–09.
    Editor, *Works of Shakespeare*.   6 vols., 1709.

    Translator, *The Life of Pythagoras* (verse only).   1707.
    Translator, with others, *Callipaedia*, by Claudius Quillet.   1712.
    Translator, with others, *Ovid's Metamorphoses*.   1717.
    Translator, *Lucan's Pharsalia*.   1718.

Reading List: *Pity and Tears: The Tragedies of Rowe* by Landon C. Burns, 1974; *Rowe and Christian Tragedy* by J. Douglas Canfield, 1977.

\*     \*     \*

Nicholas Rowe, a lawyer-turned-playwright, wrote some of the best and most frequently acted tragedies between 1700 and 1740: *Tamerlane*, *Jane Shore*, and *The Fair Penitent*. He knew Addison and Pope, and honored the theory of tragedy Pope described in his Prologue to Addison's *Cato*.

Rowe, as Shakespeare's first modern editor (1709), compared copies of the texts available to him instead of merely reprinting the First Folio, improving many obscure passages, discovering a missing scene in *Hamlet*, and adding for the first time consistent act and scene divisions, exits and entrances, and other stage directions. He demonstrated, as Alan S. Downer explains (*The British Drama: A Handbook and Brief Chronicle*), how inaccurately the Elizabethan tradition was understood 100 years later. His Preface preserves facts and traditions about Shakespeare plus observations on the way he handled various types of plays, many typical of his time, though others transcend it.

Rowe was sentimental and melodramatic in his own plays, achieving his greatest effects in pathos, though with power, in *The Fair Penitent*, *Jane Shore*, and *Lady Jane Gray*. These looked back chiefly to Thomas Otway's tender love scenes in *Venice Preserved* and *The Orphan*, and provided powerful emotional roles for actresses such as Mrs. Siddons.

Dr. Johnson, in his life of Rowe, commended Rowe's plays for interesting fables, delightful language, easily imagined domestic stories of common life, and exquisitely harmonious and appropriate diction. He declared that Lothario in *The Fair Penitent*, however, retained too much of the spectator's kindness. Rowe, borrowing *The Fair Penitent*'s plot from Massinger's *The Fatal Dowry*, has Calista seduced and abandoned by the gay Lothario (whom she really loved), married to the noble Altamount to save her honor, and reduced to utter despair when Altamount bursts in upon a love tryst and kills Lothario. Crushed by grief, she kills herself beside Lothario's coffin with her father's dagger, at his suggestion, but is tearfully received again as his daughter before she expires, thus lacing the play with Otway's pathos from a middle-class viewpoint and in the manner soon to dominate the sentimental novel.

*Tamerlane*, which demonstrated political tragedy's potential but failed to express, according to John Loftis (*The Politics of Drama in Augustan England*), the "lively conflicts embodying rival political philosophies," praised the amiable William III (Tamerlane) and attacked Louis XIV (Bajazet), and was produced annually on November 4 (William's birthday) and November 5 (the anniversary of his landing in England in 1688). Gone, however, was Marlowe's amoral Herculean superman with his boundless aspiration, love, cruelty, and wrath.

*Jane Shore*, "written in imitation of Shakespeare's style" plus much pathos, was typical of that phase of English drama (stimulated by Dryden's *All for Love*, with its love versus duty theme) when dramatists selected Shakespearean stories but developed different themes. Purportedly a Restoration heroic tragedy, the play shows political scheming as applicable to Queen Anne's time as to Elizabeth's, especially concerning Gloster, the civil war, and the uncertain succession. Richard of Gloster throws Jane, mistress to Edward IV, out into the street to starve, forbidding anyone to feed or shelter her under penalty of death. Her disguised husband saves her from rape by Lord Hastings, but the insanely jealous Alicia, Hastings's lover and Jane's close friend, pretending to appeal for Jane's banishment, substitutes a letter damning both Jane and Hastings as the crown's enemies. This prompts Gloster to execute Hastings, but drives the love-mad Alicia wild when she cannot embrace him one last time. Ironically, only Jane's still loving husband helps her, and he is taken to prison after she dies. Alicia's concluding madness recalls Otway's ending to *Venice Preserved* when Pierre and Jaffeir die on the scaffold and their ghosts appear to Belvidera, who then goes mad and dies. Rowe's handling of the Jane Shore story, the best since Shakespeare's day, advocated and applauded domestic virtue in the context of Richard of Gloster's ruthless tyranny, presenting Jane caught by as fierce a royal decree as that which tormented Sophocles' Antigone.

Rowe's last play, *Lady Jane Gray*, again focuses on a lady in distress. Though superior to the other "she-tragedies" in dramatic technique (interest is concentrated on Jane rather than being dispersed), it was never as popular. Jane, a defiant Protestant martyr, forfeits her pardon from Mary and prays from the scaffold for a monarch "To save the altars from the rage of Rome."

Nicholas Rowe helped to define a new sort of tragedy, where sympathy for love in distress and admiration for the hero's struggles against impossible odds replaced Aristotelian catharsis with its pity and terror. Characters were wept out of their evil ways; pity for the poor fallen sinners, and the implicit grim warning to others to avoid their errors, purposefully create a chasm between the tragic hero and the audience. In his best work, Rowe avoided the excesses of crass sentimentality which mars the tragedies of dramatists such as George Lillo, thus establishing his modest claim to success in tragedy.

—Louis Charles Stagg

---

**SETTLE, Elkanah.** English. Born in Dunstable, Bedfordshire, 1 February 1648. Educated at Westminster School, London; Trinity College, Oxford, matriculated 1666, but left without taking a degree. Married Mary Warner in 1673. Settled in London, 1666, and was immediately successful as a playwright; enjoyed the patronage of Rochester; involved in a literary feud with Dryden; appointed Official Poet to the City of London, 1691, and wrote the Lord Mayor's Pageants until 1708; wrote drolls for Bartholomew Fair in his old age; poor brother of the Charterhouse from 1718. *Died 12 February 1724.*

PUBLICATIONS

Plays

*Cambyses, King of Persia* (produced 1667?). 1671; revised version, 1675.
*The Empress of Morocco* (produced 1671?). 1673; edited by Bonamy Dobrée, in *Five Heroic Plays,* 1960.
*Love and Revenge,* from the play *The Fatal Contract* by William Hemmings (produced 1674). 1675.
*The Conquest of China by the Tartars* (produced 1675). 1676.
*Ibrahim the Illustrious Bassa,* from the novel by Mme. de Scudéry (produced 1676). 1677.
*Pastor Fido; or, The Faithful Shepherd,* from a play by Guarini (produced 1676). 1677.
*The Female Prelate, Pope Joan* (produced 1680). 1680.
*Fatal Love: or, The Forced Inconstancy* (produced 1680). 1680.
*The Heir of Morocco* (produced 1682). 1682.
*Distressed Innocence; or, The Princess of Persia* (produced 1690). 1691.
*The Triumphs of London* (produced 1691). 1691 (later pageants performed and published in 1692–95, 1698–1702, 1708).
*The Fairy Queen,* music by Henry Purcell, from the play *A Midsummer Night's Dream* by Shakespeare (produced 1692). 1692.
*The New Athenian Comedy.* 1693.
*The Ambitious Slave; or, A Generous Revenge* (produced 1694). 1694.
*Philaster; or, Love Lies A-Bleeding,* from the play by Beaumont and Fletcher (produced 1695). 1695.

*The World in the Moon*, music by Daniel Purcell and Jeremiah Clarke (produced 1697).   1697.

*The Virgin Prophetess; or, The Fate of Troy*, music by Gottfried Finger (produced 1701).   1701; as *Cassandra*, 1702.

*The Siege of Troy* (Bartholomew and Southwark fairs droll).   1707.

*The City-Ramble; or, A Play-House Wedding* (produced 1711).   1711.

*The Lady's Triumph*, with Lewis Theobald (produced 1718).   1718.

Fiction

*Diego Redivivus.*   1692; edited by Spiro Peterson, in *The Counterfeit Lady Unveiled*, 1961.

*The Notorious Impostor.*   2 vols., 1692; revised edition, as *The Complete Memoirs of That Notorious Impostor Will Morrell*, 1694; edited by Spiro Peterson, in *The Counterfeit Lady Unveiled*, 1961.

Verse

*Mare Clausam; or, A Ransack for the Dutch.*   1666.

*Absalom Senior; or, Achitophel Transprosed: A Poem.*   1682; edited by Harold W. Jones, in *Anti-Achitophel*, 1961.

Some 80 complimentary poems are cited in the bibliography by Frank C. Brown, below.

Other

*Notes and Observations on The Empress of Morocco Revised.*   1674.

*The Character of a Popish Successor.*   1681.

*A Defence of Dramatic Poetry.*   1698.

Editor, *Herod and Mariamne*, by Samuel Pordage.   1673.

Reading List: *Settle: His Life and Works* by Frank C. Brown, 1910 (includes bibliography).

\*     \*     \*

Faustus solicited Helen of Troy to make him immortal with a kiss. Dryden made Elkanah Settle immortal with a gibe. This very minor writer is embedded in the amber of *Absalom and Achitophel* as a fly which once buzzed around the laureate.

The facts of Settle's life are quickly told and help to explain Dryden's antagonism. Settle attended Westminster School and Trinity College, Oxford, but took no degree, setting off to seek fame and fortune in London and within a year having his first, rodomontade tragedy produced. It was pompous "in King Cambyses' vein" and indeed was called *Cambyses, King of Persia*. Its "bombastic grandiloquence" echoed Thomas Preston's tragedy of the same name (1569) and was calculated to appeal to the self-important young lawyers of Lincoln's Inn, then much impressed with the fad of heroic drama. Full of sound and fury, Settle's tyro effort threatened to eclipse Dryden and Sir Robert Howard's *Indian Emperor*.

Dryden was in the ascendant. Soon he was to become Poet Laureate and Historiographer Royal. He was to score in the theatre with *Tyrannic Love; or, The Royal Martyr* (1669) and *The Conquest of Granada* (1670). But he was doing it on his own. Settle was set up as his rival by John Wilmot, Earl of Rochester. Settle's *Empress of Morocco* was played at Whitehall by lords and ladies and was a resounding success. The Duke of Buckingham and some of his smart friends pilloried Dryden as Bayes in *The Rehearsal*, a satiric swipe at the "heroic" plays of Davenant and Dryden which must have hurt Dryden. Settle's public success was used as another club with which to beat Dryden.

After 1675 Settle lost some of his backers but little of his public. Recruited to the Whig faction by the Earl of Shaftesbury, Settle entered the pamphlet wars and attacked Dryden's interests from many angles; when Dryden turned Catholic, Settle was hired by Shaftesbury to write a "pope-burning" pageant. Settle's career stretched from 1673 into the next century and ended with his writing and performing drolls for Bartholomew Fair. Meanwhile, Dryden ticked him off as Og, while Thomas Shadwell was Doeg and held up to ridicule in *Absalom and Achitophel* and *Mac Flecknoe*.

Honestly speaking, the whole "heroic drama" was a bore and Settle's pieces are not much less bombastic than Dryden's or anyone else's. Only in *The Female Prelate*, dealing with Pope Joan, does he step really far beyond the bounds of taste in this rather tasteless period. He may have ended up in the Charterhouse while Dryden ended up in the literary Pantheon, but it was not "heroic drama" that basically explained these two extreme fates. Thomas Duffett's burlesque of *The Empress of Morocco*, clever as it is, cannot really make it sound worse than the inflated junk so cruelly pricked in *The Rehearsal*. Settle never got really much better than *The Empress of Morocco* in that unpromising genre and his operatic *Fairy Queen* (based on *A Midsummer Night's Dream*) is still remembered, albeit chiefly for the music by Henry Purcell. Settle had none of the collaborators of Dryden, nor does Settle enjoy or deserve Dryden's fame. His work was done at a time when too many plays were actually what Davenant called his 1656 entertainments at Rutland House, *Declamations and Musick*. The whole "heroic drama" was a mistake – and Settle was not even the best of that lot.

—Leonard R. N. Ashley

---

**SHADWELL, Thomas.**   English.   Born in Broomhill, Norfolk, c. 1642. Educated at home for five years, then at King Edward VI Grammar School, Bury St. Edmunds, Suffolk, 1654–56; admitted as a pensioner to Caius College, Cambridge, 1656, but left without taking a degree; entered the Middle Temple, London, 1658, and studied there for some time. Married the actress Anne Gibbs c. 1665; three sons and one daughter. Travelled abroad, then returned to London and began writing for the theatre and the opera c. 1668; involved in a feud with Dryden from 1682; succeeded Dryden as Poet Laureate and Historiographer Royal, 1689. *Died 19 November 1692.*

PUBLICATIONS

Collections

*Complete Works,* edited by Montague Summers.   5 vols., 1927.

Plays

*The Sullen Lovers; or, The Impertinents* (produced 1668).   1668.
*The Royal Shepherdess,* from the play *The Rewards of Virtue* by John Fountain (produced 1669).   1669.

*The Humorists* (produced 1670).   1671.

*Epsom Wells* (produced 1672).   1673; edited by Dorothy M. Walmsley, with *The Volunteers*, 1930.

*The Miser* (produced 1672).   1672.

*The Tempest; or, The Enchanted Island,* from the play by Shakespeare (produced 1674).   1674; edited by Christopher Spencer, in *Five Restoration Adaptations of Shakespeare,* 1965.

*The Triumphant Widow; or, The Medley of Humours,* with William Cavendish (produced 1674).   1677.

*Psyche,* music by Matthew Locke (produced 1675).   1675.

*The Libertine* (produced 1675).   1676; edited by Oscar Mandel, in *The Theatre of Don Juan,* 1963.

*The Virtuoso* (produced 1676).   1676; edited by Marjorie Hope Nicolson and David Stuart Rodes, 1966.

*A True Widow* (produced 1678).   1679.

*Timon of Athens, The Man-Hater,* from the play by Shakespeare (produced 1678).   1678.

*The Woman Captain* (produced 1679).   1680.

*The Lancashire Witches and Tegue o Divelly the Irish Priest* (produced 1681).   1682.

*The Squire of Alsatia* (produced 1688).   1688; edited by A. Norman Jeffares, in *Restoration Comedy,* 1974.

*Bury Fair* (produced 1689).   1689.

*The Amorous Bigot, with the Second Part of Tegue o Divelly* (produced 1690).   1690.

*The Scourers* (produced 1690).   1691.

*The Volunteers; or, The Stock Jobbers* (produced 1692).   1693; edited by Dorothy M. Walmsley, with *Epsom Wells,* 1930.


Verse

*The Medal of John Bayes: A Satire Against Folly and Knavery.*   1682.

*A Lenten Prologue.*   1683.

*The Tenth Satire of Juvenal.*   1687.

*A Congratulatory Poem on His Highness the Prince of Orange His Coming into England.*   1689.

*A Congratulatory Poem to the Most Illustrious Queen Mary upon Her Arrival in England.*   1689.

*Ode on the Anniversary of the King's Birth.*   1690.

*Ode to the King, on His Return from Ireland.*   1690(?).

*Votum Perenne: A Poem to the King on New Year's Day.*   1692.

*Ode on the King's Birthday.*   1692.


Other

*Notes and Observations on The Empress of Morocco by Settle,* with Dryden and John Crowne.   1674.

*Some Reflections upon the Pretended Parallel in the Play The Duke of Guise.*   1683.


Reading List: *Shadwell: His Life and Comedies* by Albert S. Borgman, 1928; *Shadwell* by Michael W. Alssid, 1967; *The Drama of Shadwell* by Don Kunz, 1972.

*       *       *

Thomas Shadwell is best known today as the target of John Dryden's satiric poem *Mac Flecknoe* (1678). Reading this cunning, exquisitely amusing lampoon, one is utterly convinced that Shadwell was no more than a clumsy, dull, nonsensical dramatist who repeated the same formula in play after play like one of his own comic humours. But reading Shadwell's drama beside Dryden's, one make a fairer assessment: while Shadwell was not nearly as accomplished a poet as his rival Dryden, he was a skillful and successful playwright. Actually, Dryden was able to enjoy a dramatic triumph over Shadwell only in the extravagantly imaginative fiction of his own poetic satire. The facts are that Shadwell was a very prolific, shrewdly professional, and highly popular Restoration dramatist.

Shadwell wrote during a literary epoch familiar to most of us either through Dryden's poetry or through some dozen outstanding plays written by a handful of gentlemen amateurs and companions to Charles II – men like the Second Duke of Buckingham, Sir Charles Sedley, Sir George Etherege, and William Wycherley. Like Dryden, Shadwell consorted with this group of witty courtiers, but he was a middle-class writer whose living depended increasingly more on box-office receipts than on their patronage. As a professional writer Shadwell was compelled to engage in nearly constant experimentation with a variety of dramatic kinds in order to appeal to an audience hungry for novelty. For example, his first play, *The Sullen Lovers*, was clearly a comedy of humours written in imitation of Ben Jonson, who along with Shakespeare had undergone a successful revival in the newly reopened theatres after Charles II's restoration to the throne. However, by the time he wrote *Epsom Wells*, Shadwell had already mastered the more modern, sophisticated comedy of wit made popular by Sedley and Etherege. Similarly, as spectacular operatic performances came into vogue, Shadwell adapted *The Tempest* and the story of Psyche; when his audience clamored for bombastic heroic tragedy, for which Dryden had created a following, Shadwell produced *The Libertine* and *Timon of Athens*. Later when political turmoil made it impossible to stage anything but farce and propaganda, Shadwell obliged with *The Woman Captain* and *The Lancashire Witches*. And when the taste was for sentimental comedy, he offered *The Squire of Alsatia* and *Bury Fair*.

Altogether between 1668 and 1692 Shadwell wrote at least eighteen plays. According to his editor, Montague Summers, some of these, like *Epsom Wells*, merited command performances at court; others, like *The Tempest*, set records for box-office receipts; fifteen of his plays continued to be performed after 1700 and six of them compiled distinguished stage histories, remaining in repertory for forty to eighty years. It was a living.

The remarkable variety in the canon of a professional playwright like Shadwell does much to dispel the common notion that Restoration drama consists essentially of heroic plays and comedies of wit. Similarly, reading Shadwell results in further correction of the gradually waning Victorian hypothesis that Restoration drama is noteworthy principally for its licentiousness and trivial frivolity. Despite their sometimes irreverent tone and frothy surface Shadwell's plays have a consistently orthodox Christian moral core; and, although they may go to extravagant lengths to entertain, invariably some socially utilitarian message is worked out in the dramatic action. His artistic credo is stated succinctly in his prologue to *The Lancashire Witches*: "Instruction is an honest Poet's aim,/And not a large or wide, but a good Fame." Among his contemporaries Shadwell enjoyed both. And sometimes envy as well.

Most of Shadwell's poetry was written in connection with his drama. He composed satiric prologues and epilogues notable for their wit and verve, their rapidly shifting tone and perspective, and their ingenious metaphors defining the playwright's relationship to his audience and plays – conceits which ranged anywhere from depicting the author as a warrior on a battlefield to a procurer in a bawdy-house. His songs typically treat of love or drinking, hunting or war; ensconced in the plays, they work to develop character or amplify theme in addition to providing a seemingly impromptu entertainment. His best poetry displays his natural ability as a dramatist: amusing characterizations, a swiftly developing argument, and clever turns of phrase.

The remainder of Shadwell's poetry consists of vituperative, Juvenalian invective like *The*

*Medal of John Bayes* or lavish panegyrics on public figures. His most conventional and unimaginative poetry was written in fulfillment of his duty as Poet Laureate – a post in which he succeeded Dryden in 1689 and served until his death in 1692. These official birthday odes, celebrations of monarchical arrivals, and congratulations for battlefield victories are frankly dull enough to have been written by Mac Flecknoe. But once again in poetry as well as drama Shadwell is notable for his range from the crude and scurrilous to the elegant and highly stylized.

Unquestionably Shadwell's real talent was for dramatic satire and comedy – pieces like *Epsom Wells*, *The Virtuoso*, and *The Squire of Alsatia*. These seem to have been inspired by a volatile combination of mischief, social purpose, and exuberant delight at the folly surrounding him. Quite likely the rest was composed because a patron or playhouse wanted it or because a reputation needed living up to or because he needed the money. This is to say that such hack work was a practical necessity, making possible that drama which is the principal justification of Shadwell's career.

—Don Kunz

---

**SHERIDAN, Richard Brinsley (Butler).**    Irish.    Born in Dublin, 30 October 1751; moved with his family to Bath, 1770. Educated at Harrow School, Middlesex, 1762–68; Waltham Abbey School, 1772–73; Middle Temple, London, 1773. Married 1) Elizabeth Ann Linley in 1773 (died, 1792), one son; 2) Esther Jane Ogle in 1795, one son. Part-owner and Director of the Drury Lane Theatre, London, 1776; served in Parliament, first as Member for Stafford, then Westminster, then Ilchester, 1780–1812: Under-Secretary of State for Foreign Affairs in the Rockingham Administration, 1782, and Secretary of the Treasury in the coalition ministry, 1783; manager of the Warren Hastings trial by Parliament, 1788–94; Treasurer of the Navy, 1806; Member of the Privy Council. *Died 7 July 1816.*

PUBLICATIONS

Collections

> *Works*, edited by F. Stainworth.   1874.
> *Plays and Poems*, edited by R. Crompton Rhodes.   3 vols., 1928.
> *Letters*, edited by Cecil Price.   3 vols., 1966.
> *Dramatic Works*, edited by Cecil Price.   2 vols., 1973.

Plays

> *The Rivals* (produced 1775).   1775; edited by R. L. Purdy, 1935.
> *St. Patrick's Day; or, The Scheming Lieutenant* (produced 1775).   1788.
> *The Duenna*, music by Thomas Linley and others (produced 1775).   1775.
> *A Trip to Scarborough*, from the play *The Relapse* by Vanbrugh (produced 1777).   1781.

*The School for Scandal* (produced 1777).   1780.

*The Camp,* music by Thomas Linley (produced 1778).   1795.

*The Critic; or, A Tragedy Rehearsed* (produced 1779).   1781.

*The Storming of Fort Omoa* (interlude in *Harlequin Fortunatus* by Henry Woodward; produced 1780).

*Robinson Crusoe; or, Harlequin Friday,* music by Thomas Linley (produced 1781).   Songs published 1781.

*The Glorious First of June,* with James Cobb (benefit entertainment, produced 1794).   Songs published 1794; revised version, as *Cape St. Vincent* (produced 1797), songs published 1797.

*The Stranger,* from a translation by Benjamin Thompson of a play by Kotzebue (produced 1798).

*Pizarro,* from a play by Kotzebue (produced 1799).   1799.

*The Forty Thieves,* with Charles Ward and Colman the Younger, music by Michael Kelly (produced 1806).   1808; as *Ali Baba,* 1814.

Verse

*The Ridotto of Bath: A Panegyric.*   1771.

*The Love Epistle of Aristaenetus,* with Nathaniel Halhed.   1771.

*The Rival Beauties,* with Miles Peter Andrews(?).   1772.

*Verses to the Memory of Garrick.*   1779; as *The Tears of Genius,* 1780.

Other

*A Familiar Epistle to the Author of the Epistle to William Chambers.*   1774.

*Speeches.*   5 vols., 1816.

Bibliography: in *Plays and Poems,* 1928.

Reading List: *Sheridan* (biography) by Walter S. Sichel, 2 vols., 1909; *Harlequin Sheridan: The Man and the Legends* by R. Crompton Rhodes, 1933; *Sheridan of Drury Lane* by Alice Glasgow, 1940; *Sheridan* by Lewis Gibbs, 1947; *Sheridan and Kotzebue: A Comparative Essay* by G. Sinko, 1949; *Sheridan: The Track of a Comet* by Madeleine Bingham, 1972; *Sheridan's Comedies: Their Contexts and Achievements* by Mark S. Auburn, 1977; *Sheridan and the Drama of Georgian England* by John Loftis, 1977.

\*     \*     \*

Sheridan's first comedy, *The Rivals,* was produced in 1775, as were *St. Patrick's Day; or, The Scheming Lieutenant,* a farce, and *The Duenna,* a comic opera. *The Duenna* made his name. Then he adapted Vanbrugh's *The Relapse* (1696) to suit the greater refinement of his own age and called it *A Trip to Scarborough*; it was staged in February 1777, and followed in the same year by *The School for Scandal*; two years later came *The Critic.* With the exception of *Pizarro,* which he adapted from the German of Kotzebue in 1799, and some minor work, his dramatic career was compressed into four years.

*The Rivals* is characterized by liveliness and vitality. The plot is skilfully devised, the dialogue is fresh, and the characters, though types, are well differentiated and probably created with particular actors and actresses in mind, for Sheridan knew about the theatre from an early age: his father was an actor and the author of a successful farce as well as a teacher of elocution, and his mother had written successful comedies. Sheridan set the action of *The Rivals* in Bath, where his father had set up his school of elocution in 1770, and where his own youth had been socially successful. He danced and flirted and observed the fashionable life of this elegant spa, with its concerts, plays, and balls, its circulating libraries, cards, and scandal occupying the time of the people of distinction who frequented it. He captured its ethos well in *The Rivals*. One heroine, Lydia Languish, headlong and romantic, derives much of her silliness from her diet of light reading, and the other, Julia Melville, is sentimental in the eighteenth-century manner. Jack Absolute refuses his father's plans for him until he finds that the girl chosen is Lydia whom he loves – but there is the complication that he has pretended to be Ensign Beverley, to cater to Lydia's romantic nature. Jack's relationship with his autocratic father adds to the play's liveliness, but the other hero, Faulkland, who suffers from jealousy, can seem sickly to a modern audience in his fashionably sentimental speeches to Julia. But Sir Lucius O'Trigger, the fire-eating Irishman, and Mrs. Malaprop, vulgar, ambitious, a magnificent mishandler of language, give the play its own particular comic – and farcical – flavour. Vitality and speed of action have kept this play successful on the stage.

*The School for Scandal* is more serious, for Sheridan was satirising the excesses of contemporary journalism and scandal-mongering. But what he created in his mockery of the polite world of his own day was lasting comedy. He used proven ingredients, lovers kept apart and finally rewarded, mistaken identity, the country girl out of her depth in the life of the town, the reassessment of an apparent rake, and, above all, the exposure – and, significantly, the explanation – of hypocrisy. It is all done very effectively, with sparkling conversation, a clever, indeed complex, plot of intrigue, a comedy of manners which exposes the soulful sentimentality of contemporary drama, the slandering, the malice, selfishness, and hypocrisy of contemporary society. Sheridan's ironies are clear: he distinguished between appearance and reality brilliantly, without the coarseness or indeed the immorality of Restoration comedy; he supplied suspense, the ludicrous situation, the unexpected reversal; he knew what kept – and still keeps – an audience amused. And so the contrast between the Surface brothers, the effect of the screen's falling upon the main characters, the reconciliation of Sir Peter and Lady Teazle, the marriage of Charles and Maria are all timeless in achievement.

Sheridan's views of comedy emerge not only in the second prologue to *The Rivals* but in *The Critic*, which was inspired by Buckingham's *The Rehearsal*. In it he mocked his contemporary Cumberland in the character of Sir Fretful Plagiary, and contemporary critics in the characters Puff and Sneer. This play is an amusing parody of contemporary dramatic techniques, which were often fairly crude – and so there are often references which are obscure to modern audiences or readers. *The Critic* is in effect a series of sketches, designed as an after-play to *Hamlet* – hence when Tilburina burlesques Ophelia's speech the audiences would have had the original in mind. Sheridan is exposing dull dialogue, artificial devices and asides, the melodrama inherent in plots which were unsophisticatedly resolved, the insistence upon fashion in dress, stereotyped delivery of lines, and crude acting in badly illuminated auditoriums. In fact, he is giving us a somewhat exasperated manager's view of the unsatisfactory elements of the stage in his own day: but he does it, as usual, with the light touch and sense of absurdity which illuminate all his own drama.

—A. Norman Jeffares

---

**SOUTHERNE, Thomas.**   Irish.   Born in Oxmantown, near Dublin, in Autumn 1660. Educated at Trinity College, Dublin (pensioner), 1676–78, M.A. 1696; entered the Middle Temple, London, 1678. Served as an Ensign in Princess Anne's Regiment, and rose to the command of a company, 1685–88. Thereafter devoted himself entirely to writing for the stage, at first as a protégé and disciple of Dryden; retired in 1726. *Died 22 May 1746.*

PUBLICATIONS

Collections

> *Plays,* edited by T. Evans.   3 vols., 1774.

Plays

> *The Loyal Brother; or The Persian Prince* (produced 1682).   1682; edited by P. Hamelius, 1911.
> *The Disappointment; or, The Mother in Fashion* (produced 1684).   1684.
> *Sir Anthony Love; or, The Rambling Lady* (produced 1690).   1691.
> *The Wives' Excuse; or, Cuckolds Make Themselves* (produced 1691).   1692; edited by Ralph R. Thornton, 1973.
> *The Maid's Last Prayer; or, Any, Rather Than Fail* (produced 1693).   1693; edited by Ralph R. Thornton, 1978.
> *The Fatal Marriage; or, The Innocent Adultery,* from the story "The Nun" by Aphra Behn (produced 1694).   1694.
> *Oroonoko,* from the story by Aphra Behn (produced 1695).   1696; edited by Maximillian E. Novak and David Stuart Rodes, 1976.
> *The Fate of Capua* (produced 1700).   1700.
> *The Spartan Dame* (produced 1719).   1719.
> *Money the Mistress* (produced 1726).   1726.

Reading List: *Southerne, Dramatist* by John W. Dobbs, 1933; *The Comedy of Manners* by Kenneth Muir, 1970.

\*       \*       \*

Thomas Southerne's career as a dramatist was, like his life's span, a lengthy one. His first play, *The Loyal Brother,* a panegyric to the Duke of York, appeared in the troubled year 1682; his last, *Money the Mistress,* a failed comedy, in 1726. His major works came apace between 1690 and 1696: three comedies in the manners genre and two extraordinarily popular tragedies in the pathetic vein.

Of the comedies, *Sir Anthony Love* was best received; its success gave rise to a new practice, the author's sixth-night benefit. The action is conventionally vigorous, the intrigues multiplex; Southerne's twist lies in representing his rake-hero, Sir Anthony, by "the female Montford bare above the knee." The next comedy, *The Wives' Excuse,* a flat failure, paradoxically excites critical interest today as the link between the older plays of Etherege and Wycherley and the revival of the manners genre by Congreve and Vanbrugh. The foibles of fashionable Londoners are exhaustively chronicled, but the play devolves into a "problem play" with its distressed heroine consciously choosing not to take the usual revenge on an impertinent coxcomb of a husband. Stung by the failure, Southerne reverted to the sure-fire formula of gallantry and intrigue in *The Maid's Last Prayer,* adding genuinely comic (nigh farcical) scenes of amateur "musick-meetings," Lady Susan's dogged pursuit of men, any man, rather than fail, and, curiously, one of the darkest scenes of sexual revenge in dramatic literature.

The success of *The Fatal Marriage* and *Oroonoko* confirmed Southerne's popular reputation in his own generation. Adapting both plots from the works of Aphra Behn, Southerne commingled new action and characters, as well as counterpoint comic sub-plots, to accentuate the pathos and distressed nobility of his sentimentalized tragic protagonists. Each play remained an actor's vehicle well into the nineteenth century, Garrick having altered *The Fatal Marriage* in 1757 to *Isabella*.

Of the remaining plays, *The Disappointment* is an olio of dramatic elements; it points, however, to an interest in the distressed-heroine problem play. *The Fate of Capua*, a neo-classical tragedy set in the Second Punic War, was unsuccessful, despite moving individual scenes. *The Spartan Dame* was Southerne's true valedictory to the theatre, though it was really an old play, having been largely completed in 1687 but denied production because of its fable (from Plutarch) – usurpation by a daughter.

In a partisan age, Southerne managed to maintain widespread and abiding friendships: Dryden, Wycherley, Congreve, Dennis, Gildon, the Earls of Orrery; later Pope and his circle regarded him with affection; his literary mid-wifery to unproduced dramatists was legendary; and his dedications to Whigs or Tories were made with an eye to profit, not politics. In the theatre, Southerne's astute eye caught the changes in the audiences' taste and composition; he learned early to supply these new arbiters of the box and pit with drama of pathos – she-tragedies – not the out-of-style realistic, satiric comedy. Therein his popularity lay.

—Ralph R. Thornton

---

**STEELE, Sir Richard.** Irish. Born in Dublin, baptized 12 March 1672. Educated at Charterhouse, London, where he met Joseph Addison, 1684–89; matriculated at Christ Church, Oxford, 1690; postmaster at Merton College, Oxford, 1691–94, but left without taking a degree. Enlisted as a cadet in the Duke of Ormonde's guards, 1694; Ensign in Lord Cutts's Regiment, 1695, and served as Cutts's confidential secretary, 1696–97; Captain, stationed at the Tower of London, by 1700; transferred as Captain to Lord Lucas's Regiment in 1702. Married 1) Margaret Ford Stretch in 1705 (died, 1706); 2) Mary Scurlock in 1707 (died, 1718), two sons and two daughters. Wrote extensively for the theatre, 1701–05; Gentleman-Writer to Prince George of Denmark, 1706–08; Gazetteer (i.e., Manager of the *Gazette*, the official government publication), 1707–10; Commissioner of Stamps, 1710–13; Founding Editor, *The Tatler*, to which Addison was the major contributor, 1709–11; Founder, and Editor with Addison, *The Spectator*, 1711–12; Founding Editor, *The Guardian*, 1713; elected Member of Parliament for Stockbridge, Hampshire, 1713, but expelled for anti-government views; Founding Editor, *The Englishman*, 1713–14, *The Lover*, 1714, and *The Reader*, 1714; on accession of George I, 1714, appointed Justice of the Peace, Deputy Lieutenant for the County of Middlesex, Surveyor of the Royal Stables at Hampton Court, and Supervisor of the Drury Lane Theatre, London: granted life patent of Drury Lane, 1715; Member of Parliament for Boroughbridge, Yorkshire, 1715; Founding Editor, *Town Talk*, 1715–16, *The Tea-Table*, and *Chit-Chat*, 1716; appointed Commissioner for Forfeited Estates in Scotland, 1716; quarrelled with Addison, 1719; Founding Editor, *The Plebeian*, 1719, and *The Theatre*, 1720; Member of Parliament for Wendover, Buckinghamshire, 1722; retired to Wales, 1724. Knighted, 1715. *Died 1 September 1729.*

PUBLICATIONS

### Collections

*Correspondence,* edited by R. Blanchard.    1941; revised edition, 1968.
*Plays,* edited by Shirley S. Kenny.    1971.

### Plays

*The Funeral; or, Grief a-la-Mode* (produced 1701).    1702.
*The Lying Lover; or, The Ladies' Friendship* (produced 1703).    1704.
*The Tender Husband; or, The Accomplished Fools* (produced 1703).    1705.
*The Conscious Lovers* (produced 1722).    1723.

### Verse

*The Procession: A Poem on Her Majesty's Funeral.*    1695.
*Occasional Verse,* edited by R. Blanchard.    1952.

### Other

*The Christian Hero, An Argument Proving That No Principles But Those of Religion Are Sufficient to Make a Great Man.*    1701; edited by R. Blanchard, 1932.
*The Tatler,* with Addison.    4 vols., 1710–11; edited by G. A. Aitken, 4 vols., 1898–99; selections edited by L. Gibbs, 1953.
*The Spectator,* with Addison.    8 vols., 1712–15; edited by D. F. Bond, 5 vols., 1965; selections edited by R. J. Allen, 1957.
*An Englishman's Thanks to the Duke of Marlborough.*    1712.
*A Letter to Sir M. W[arton] Concerning Occasional Peers.*    1713.
*The Importance of Dunkirk.*    1713.
*The Guardian,* with others.    2 vols., 1714; edited by Alexander Chalmers, 1802.
*The Englishman* (2 series, and an epistle).    3 vols., 1714–16; edited by R. Blanchard, 1955.
*The Crisis, with Some Seasonable Remarks on the Danger of a Popish Successor.*    1714.
*The French Faith Represented in the Present State of Dunkirk.*    1714.
*A Letter Concerning the Bill for Preventing the Growth of Schism.*    1714.
*Mr. Steele's Apology for Himself and His Writings.*    1714.
*A Letter from the Earl of Mar to the King.*    1715.
*A Letter Concerning the Condemned Lords.*    1716.
*Account of Mr. Desagulier's New-Invented Chimneys.*    1716.
*An Account of the Fish Pool,* with Joseph Gillmore.    1718.
*The Joint and Humble Address to the Tories and Whigs Concerning the Intended Bill of Peerage.*    1719.
*A Letter to the Earl of O—d Concerning the Bill of Peerage.*    1719.
*The Plebeian.*    1719; edited by R. Hurd, in Addison's *Works,* 1856.
*The Spinster, in Defence of the Woollen Manufactures.*    1719.
*The Crisis of Property.*    1720.
*A Nation a Family; or, A Plan for the Improvement of the South-Sea Proposal.*    1720.
*The State of the Case Between the Lord Chamberlain and the Governor of the Royal Company of Comedians.*    1720.

*The Theatre.*    1720; edited by John Loftis, 1962.
*Tracts and Pamphlets,* edited by R. Blanchard.    1944.
*Steele's Periodical Journalism 1714–16: The Lover, The Reader, Town Talk, Chit-Chat,*
edited by R. Blanchard.    1959.

Editor, *The Ladies Library.*    3 vols., 1714.
Editor, *Poetical Miscellanies.*    1714.

Reading List: *Steele* by Willard Connely, 1934; *Steele at Drury Lane* by John Loftis, 1952; *Steele, Addison, and Their Periodical Essays* by Arthur R. Humphreys, 1959; *Steele: The Early Career,* 1964, and *The Later Career,* 1970, both by Calhoun Winton.

\*      \*      \*

Though best remembered as a periodical essayist, Sir Richard Steele began his literary career in the theatre – if, that is, one forgets and forgives his moralizing tract *The Christian Hero,* an unsuccessful attempt at self-admonition. His plays were frank attempts to make piety more palatable, while avoiding the sexual excesses for which Collier had condemned the stage, and which increasingly middle-class audiences were also finding offensive.

The first, *The Funeral,* has several touches of originality, notably in its satire on the undertaking business, its sprightly yet sympathetic treatment of its female characters, and its liveliness of plotting. Indeed, two of the participants in Gildon's *A Comparison Between the Two Stages* allege that in this latter respect the play resembles a farce more than it does a comedy, and it may be regretted that Steele never successfully evaded formal considerations of this kind – though two fragments, *The School of Action* and *The Gentleman,* do begin to assert the kind of freedom from the rules that Gay and Fielding more happily achieved.

*The Lying Lover* was unalleviated by realism, displayed less comic spirit, and was, as Steele ruefully admitted, "damn'd for its piety." Loosely derived from Corneille's *Le Menteur,* it features a pathetic repentance scene, in which its hero, Young Bookwit, awakens in prison to find that he has killed a rival in a drunken duel. For this he is duly contrite in blank verse, to the extent of putting forgiveness before honour. There is some wit in the quixotic Bookwit's romancing in the earlier scenes, and his respectful welcome to Newgate by his fellow inmates hints at the inverted morality of *The Beggar's Opera:* yet, just a few scenes later, Steele perpetrates a double shift in the plot, lacking any sense of its own fatal absurdity.

*The Tender Husband,* Steele's third play, also proved to be his last to reach the stage for nearly eighteen years. It has a female Quixote, or prototype Lydia Languish, as its heroine – and, indeed, the original of Tony Lumpkin in that heroine's cousin, Humphry Gubbin. Unfortunately, the sub-plot featuring the titular husband, who devises an unlikely test of his wife's faithfulness by disguising his own mistress as a suitor, disrupts the comic flow, and complicates the conclusion with a sentimental reconciliation.

In the following years, Steele was increasingly active as a Whig politician, his major literary achievement being, of course, the succession of periodicals he created, some written in collaboration with Joseph Addison. Of these, the best remembered are *The Tatler, The Spectator,* and *The Guardian,* with the irrelevantly titled *The Theatre* probably the most important of the later series. Whether or not Steele succeeded in his aim "to make the pulpit, the bar, and the stage all act in concert in the cause of piety, justice, and virtue" is arguable: but he certainly perfected a distinctive new form of clubable *belles lettres,* incidentally exploring techniques of characterization for his recurrent *personae* which were to be of significance to the early novelists, and publishing some first-rate dramatic criticism.

Although *The Conscious Lovers,* which did not reach the stage until 1722, was influential in the development of the *comédie larmoyante* in France, to the modern mind it merely demonstrates that, at its most sentimental, eighteenth-century comedy was no laughing matter. With the exception of its scenes below stairs – their purpose all too evidently to sugar a didactic pill – it is a distinctly unfunny play: yet, according to Steele, an audience's pleasure might be "too exquisite for laughter," and thus better expressed in the tears evoked by the inexpressibly virtuous behaviour of his hero, Young Bevil, and by the convenient reshufflings of the characters in the closing scene.

The mercantile morality of the play is at once over-explicit and interruptive, and its characters are in neither the humours nor the manners tradition, but mere ethical absolutes. No wonder that Fielding's Parson Adams considered it the first play fit for a Christian to read since the pagan tragedies – but then good Parson Adams lacked both irony and a sense of incongruity, as does *The Conscious Lovers*. Steele is better remembered by the feeling for both irony *and* incongruity in his earlier plays, and, of course, by his largeness of heart as a periodical essayist.

—Simon Trussler

---

**TATE, Nahum.** Irish. Born Nahum Teate in Dublin in 1652. Educated at Trinity College, Dublin, 1668–72, B.A. 1672. Settled in London, 1672; began writing for the theatre, 1678; also subsequently involved in extensive work as editor and translator of various authors; Editor, with M. Smith, *The Monitor*, 1713; appointed Poet Laureate, 1692, and Historiographer Royal, 1702. *Died 30 July 1715.*

PUBLICATIONS

Plays

> *Brutus of Alba; or, The Enchanted Lovers* (produced 1678).    1678.
> *The Loyal General* (produced 1679).    1680.
> *King Richard the Second*, from the play by Shakespeare.    1681; as *The Sicilian Usurper* (produced 1680), 1691; as *The Tyrant of Sicily* (produced 1681).
> *King Lear*, from the play by Shakespeare (produced 1681).    1681; edited by James Black, 1975.
> *The Ingratitude of a Commonwealth; or, The Fall of Caius Martius Coriolanus*, from the play by Shakespeare (produced 1681).    1682.
> *A Duke and No Duke*, from the play *Trappolin Supposed a Prince* by Aston Cokayne (produced 1684).    1685; edited by Leo A. Hughes and Arthur H. Scouten, in *Ten English Farces*, 1948.
> *Cuckold's Haven; or, An Alderman No Conjuror*, from the play *Eastward Ho* by Jonson, Chapman, and Marston (produced 1685).    1685.
> *The Island Princess*, from the play by Fletcher (produced 1687).    1687.
> *Dido and Aeneas*, music by Henry Purcell (produced 1689).    1690; edited by G. A. Macfarren, 1841.
> *Injured Love; or, The Cruel Husband.*    1707.

## Verse

*Poems.*   1677; revised edition, 1684.
*The Second Part of Absalom and Achitophel,* with Dryden.   1682.
*On the Sacred Memory of Our Late Sovereign.*   1685.
*A Pastoral in Memory of the Duke of Ormonde.*   1688.
*A Poem Occasioned by His Majesty's Voyage to Holland.*   1691.
*A Poem Occasioned by the Late Discontents.*   1691.
*Characters of Virtue and Vice, Attempted in Verse from a Treatise by Joseph
    Hall.*   1691.
*An Ode upon Her Majesty's Birthday.*   1693.
*A Present for the Ladies.*   1693.
*A Poem upon the Late Promotion of Several Eminent Persons.*   1694.
*In Memory of Joseph Washington: An Elegy.*   1694.
*An Ode upon the University of Dublin's Foundation.*   1694.
*Mausolaeum: A Funeral Poem on Our Late Queen.*   1695.
*An Elegy on the Late Archbishop of Canterbury.*   1695.
*The Anniversary Ode for His Majesty's Birthday.*   1698.
*A Consolatory Poem to Lord Cutts.*   1698.
*Elegies.*   1699.
*An Essay of a Character of Sir George Treby.*   1700.
*Funeral Poems.*   1700.
*Panacea: A Poem upon Tea.*   1700; as *A Poem upon Tea,* 1702.
*An Elegy in Memory of Ralph Marshall.*   1700.
*A Congratulatory Poem on the New Parliament.*   1701.
*The Kentish Worthies.*   1701.
*A Monumental Poem in Memory of Sir George Treby.*   1702.
*Portrait-Royal: A Poem upon Her Majesty's Picture.*   1703.
*The Song for New Year's Day.*   1703.
*The Triumph: A Poem on the Glorious Successes of the Last Year.*   1705.
*Britannia's Prayer for the Queen.*   1706.
*The Triumph of Union.*   1707.
*A Congratulatory Poem to Prince George of Denmark.*   1708.
*The Muse's Memorial to the Earl of Oxford.*   1712.
*The Muses Bower.*   1713.
*The Triumph of Peace.*   1713.
*A Poem Sacred to the Memory of Queen Anne.*   1714.

## Other

*An Essay for Promoting of Psalmody.*   1710.

Editor, *Poems by Several Hands.*   1685.
Editor, *A Memorial for the Learned,* by J. D.   1686.
Editor, *The Life of Alexander the Great,* by Quintus Curtius Rufius.   1690.
Editor, *The Political Anatomy of Ireland,* by Sir William Petty.   1691.
Editor, *Guzman,* by Roger Boyle.   1693.
Editor, *The Four Epistles of A. G. Bushbequius.*   1694.
Editor, *Miscellanea Sacra; or, Poems on Divine and Moral Subjects.*   1696; revised
    edition, 1698.
Editor, *An Essay on Poetry,* by John Sheffield, Duke of Buckingham.   1697.
Editor, *The Original of the Soul* (Nosce Teipsum), by Sir John Davies.   1697.
Editor, *The Innocent Epicure; or, The Art of Angling,* by J. S.   1697.

Translator, with others, *Ovid's Epistles*.  1680.

Translator, *Syphilus: A Poetical History of the French Disease*, by Fracastoro.  1686.

Translator, with "a person of quality," *The Aethiopian History*, by Heliodorus.  1686; as *The Triumphs of Love and Constancy*, 1687.

Translator, with others, *Cowley's Six Books of Plants*.  1689.

Translator, *The Life of the Prince of Condé*.  2 vols., 1693.

Translator, with others, *The Satires of Juvenal*, with *The Satires of Persius* translated by Dryden.  1693.

Translator, with Nicholas Brady, *An Essay of a New Version of the Psalms of David*.  1695; revised edition, 1695, 1696; *Supplement*, 1700.

Translator, *Majesta Imperii Britannici, The Glories of Great Britain*, by Mr. Maidwell.  1706.

Translator, with Aaron Hill, *The Celebrated Speeches of Ajax and Ulysses*, by Ovid.  1708.

Translator, with others, *The Works of Lucian*.  4 vols., 1710–11.

Translator, with others, *Ovid's Art of Love and His Remedy of Love*.  1712.

Reading List: *Tate* by Christopher Spencer, 1972.

*     *     *

Nahum Tate is best known for his scaled-down version of *King Lear* with its love story between Cordelia and Edgar and its happy ending in which Lear retires and leaves his kingdom to the lovers. After Tate's version was finally replaced in the theatre by Shakespeare's in 1838, the word "Tatefication" was coined to refer to the debasement of great literary works; however, the term ignores the ingenuity with which the adaptation was fitted to the Restoration theatre and its long success. The farce *A Duke and No Duke* (based on Aston Cokayne's *Trappolin Supposed a Prince*, 1633) also continued to please audiences until well into the 19th century; for the second edition (1693) Tate wrote an extended defence of farce. Tate's libretto for Henry Purcell's operatic masterpiece *Dido and Aeneas* contains verse that, though undistinguished as poetry, is well designed for setting to music.

Tate was not a vigorous or original writer, and his best work was done in adaptation, translation, or collaboration. He joined successfully with Dryden in Ovid's *Epistles* and Juvenal's *Satires*, as well as *The Second Part of Absalom and Achitophel* (1682). With a clerical family background and experience in translation and in writing for music, Tate was well-qualified to collaborate with Nicholas Brady in versifying the Psalms. Their *New Version of the Psalms of David* was more polished and elegant than the old Sternhold and Hopkins version of 1562, and was generally used in Anglican churches for more than a century. Some of the Tate-Brady renderings are included as hymns in modern hymnals, e.g., "Thro' All the Changing Scenes of Life" (Psalm 34) and "As Pants the Hart for Cooling Streams" (Psalm 62). The carol "While Shepherds Watched Their Flocks by Night" first appeared in the *Supplement to the New Version*.

Of the 102 poems in Tate's two collections (1677, 1684), many are on melancholy themes but some suggest Cavalier or Metaphysical models or echo Shakespeare or Milton. The odes, elegies, and other occasional poems that Tate felt were a laureate's duty generally do an adequate job of expressing (sometimes to musical accompaniment by Purcell or John Blow) the grand thoughts that are appropriate for the public occasion. A more relaxed poem (perhaps his best original work) is the amusing, mock-heroic *Panacea: A Poem upon Tea*.

—Christopher Spencer

**VANBRUGH, Sir John.** English. Born in London, baptized 24 January 1664. Educated at the King's School, Chester, to age 19; also studied in France, 1683–85. Commissioned ensign in the 13th foot regiment of Lord Huntingdon, 1686; arrested in Calais for espionage, and imprisoned in France, 1688–92; Captain in Lord Berkeley's Marine Regiment, 1696; Captain in Lord Huntingdon's Regiment, 1702. Married Henrietta Maria Yarborough in 1719; one son. Architect: designed Castle Howard, 1701, Haymarket Theatre, 1703, Blenheim Palace, 1705, Fleurs (Floors Castle), 1716, Seaton Delavel, 1720, etc.; Comptroller to the Public Works, 1702–13, 1715; Manager, with Congreve, Haymarket Theatre, London, 1705–06; appointed Carlisle Herald, 1703, and Clarenceux King-at-Arms, 1704–26, in the College of Heralds; Surveyor of Greenwich Hospital, 1715. Knighted, 1723. *Died 26 March 1726.*

PUBLICATIONS

Collections

    *Complete Works,* edited by Bonamy Dobrée and Geoffrey Webb. 4 vols., 1927–28.

Play

    *The Relapse; or, Virtue in Danger* (produced 1696). 1697; edited by Bernard Harris, 1971.
    *Aesop,* 2 parts, from a play by Boursault (produced 1696–97). 2 vols., 1697.
    *The Provoked Wife* (produced 1697). 1697; edited by Peter Dixon, 1975.
    *The Country House,* from a play by Dancourt (produced 1698). 1715.
    *The Pilgrim,* from the play by Fletcher (produced 1700). 1700.
    *The False Friend,* from a play by Le Sage (produced 1702). 1702.
    *Squire Trelooby,* with Congreve and William Walsh, from a play by Molière (produced 1704). Revised version by James Ralph published as *The Cornish Squire,* 1734.
    *The Confederacy,* from a play by Dancourt (produced 1705; also produced as *The City Wives' Confederacy).* 1705.
    *The Mistake,* from a play by Molière (produced 1705). 1706.
    *The Cuckold in Conceit* (produced 1707).
    *Plays.* 2 vols., 1719.
    *A Journey to London,* completed by Cibber (as *The Provoked Husband,* produced 1728). 1728.

Other

    *A Short Vindication of The Relapse and The Provoked Wife from Immorality and Profaneness.* 1698.
    *Vanbrugh's Justification of What He Deposed in the Duchess of Marlborough's Late Trial.* 1718.

Reading List: *Vanbrugh, Architect and Dramatist,* 1938, and *The Imagination of Vanbrugh and His Fellow Artists,* 1954, both by Laurence Whistler; *Vanbrugh* by Bernard Harris, 1967; "Vanbrugh and the Conventions of Restoration Comedy" by Gerald M. Berkowitz, in *Genre*

6, 1973; *Masks and Façades: Vanbrugh: The Man in His Setting* by Madeleine Bingham, 1974; *Vanbrugh* by Kerry Downes, 1977.

\*    \*    \*

Vanbrugh's reputation as a major comic dramatist rests on two plays produced within six months of each other at the end of the seventeenth century, *The Relapse* and *The Provok'd Wife*. Like Etherege and Wycherley, the two finest comic playwrights of the previous generation, Vanbrugh was not a professional writer and devoted only a fairly short period of his life to the theatre, so that his output, like theirs, is relatively small. Indeed he is at least as renowned for his architecture, especially Castle Howard and Blenheim Palace, as for his plays. Belonging to the generation of dramatists that includes Congreve, Farquhar, Steele, and Colley Cibber, Vanbrugh was writing after the Glorious Revolution of 1688 when the theatre was again coming under moralistic attacks because of its alleged licentiousness and obscenity. Vanbrugh himself was criticized in the most influential of these, Jeremy Collier's comprehensive *A Short View of the Immorality and Profaneness of the English Stage* (1698), and published a reply in the same year, *A Short Vindication*, in which he defends *The Relapse* and *The Provok'd Wife* against Collier's strictures. At a time when comic drama was beginning to undergo the transformation that led to the homiletic "exemplary" or "sentimental" comedy of the eighteenth century, which concentrated on providing models of virtue and examples of moral reformation to be emulated rather than on comedy's traditional function of ridiculing vice, folly, and affectation, Vanbrugh was intent on keeping alive the satirical mainstream of seventeenth-century comedy descending from Ben Jonson. Like Congreve, he was greatly indebted to the dramatists of Charles II's reign who developed the so-called "wit" or "manners" comedy of the Restoration, but because of his originality in handling its conventions he made a distinctive contribution to this kind of comedy. This is partly because of his essentially serious preoccupation with the subject of marriage, especially the tensions between husband and wife in ill-matched and unhappy relationships, and partly because of the robust energy of his plays that manifests itself in his rich characterization and his inventiveness in creating comic situations. Vanbrugh does in fact cross Shadwell's comedy of "humours" with Etherege's and Congreve's comedy of "wit." Although less caustically satirical than Wycherley, less stylistically refined than Congreve, and less genial than Farquhar, he is undoubtedly one of the wittiest of Restoration writers and for sheer vitality he has few equals among his contemporaries and eighteenth-century successors.

Vanbrugh wrote *The Relapse*, his first play to be staged, in response to Cibber's *Love's Last Shift* (1696), in which Amanda employs subterfuge and deception, including seduction, to win back her rakish husband Loveless who has deserted her. Cibber presents Amanda's reprehensible conduct as admirable, and Loveless, overwhelmed by her display of wifely love, is instantly reconciled to her and morally reformed. Vanbrugh clearly found this sentimental and sententious dénouement facile, dishonest, and unconvincing, and in *The Relapse* wrote a sequel that is also a reply to *Love's Last Shift*. *The Relapse* does, however, stand as a completely independent work that can be appreciated without reference to Cibber's considerably inferior play. Vanbrugh's main plot continues the story of Amanda and Loveless after the penitent's apparent rehabilitation and shows how temporary such reformations usually are. Loveless soon reverts to his promiscuous ways when temptation arrives in the form of Amanda's widowed cousin Berinthia, whereas the virtuous Amanda resists Worthy's offer of adulterous love. At the end of the play Vanbrugh presents no solution to the problem of Amanda and Loveless's marriage, which is left unresolved. Interesting and unusual as this part of the play is, it almost takes second place to the sub-plot concerning Lord Foppington. Vanbrugh again draws on *Love's Last Shift*, since Lord Foppington is Cibber's Sir Novelty Fashion elevated to the peerage, but Vanbrugh also transforms Cibber's amusing portrait of a fop into not only the most rounded presentation of a fashionable beau in contemporary drama but one of the great comic characters of the English stage. Almost as unforgettable is Sir Tunbelly Clumsey, Vanbrugh's version of another stereotype of Restoration comedy, the boorish country knight. Structurally *The Relapse* may be faulty, and Vanbrugh, a fundamentally moral writer, is unable to eschew completely the sentimentality that mars Cibber's play so badly, but its sustained comic brilliance more than compensates for its defects.

*The Provok'd Wife*, a better organised play than its predecessor, also contains one of the best comic characters of the period, Sir John Brute, the most memorable of the numerous husbands in Restoration comedy who are heartily sick of marriage and their wives and who try, not very successfully, to devote themselves to a life of debauchery. The surly, rude, and stubborn Sir John has ruined his marriage, and Vanbrugh explores sympathetically the predicament of Lady Brute who is maltreated by her husband but who is too virtuous to give herself to her admirer Constant. Vanbrugh deals with the issue of marital incompatibility, at a time when divorce was virtually impossible, in a sensitive and humane way, not in the flippant and jokey manner typical of contemporary comedy, and is too realistic to offer an easy theatrical solution producing a happy ending for Lady Brute. As in *The Relapse*, there is no tidy resolution of the main plot.

Apart from the unfinished *A Journey to London*, which reached the stage in 1728 in a version revised, completed, and sentimentalized by Colley Cibber entitled *The Provok'd Husband*, Vanbrugh's other dramatic works are either adaptations or translations of earlier plays. His one attempt to revamp an English play, a prose version of Fletcher's *The Pilgrim*, impoverishes rather than enriches the original, but the opposite occurs in the case of some of his translations. As a translator of recent French plays, including some of Molière's, Vanbrugh was far from slavish and felt free to alter and add to his sources, the result being that he imbued them with some of his typical vigour and broad humour. The outstanding example is *The Confederacy*, a superb adaptation of Dancourt's *Les Bourgeoises à la Mode*, itself a lively and witty comedy that Vanbrugh, by transferring the action from Paris to London, nevertheless succeeds in enhancing from beginning to end. Also worthy of note is *Aesop*, based on Boursault's *Les Fables d'Ésope*, in which Vanbrugh characteristically tones down the sentiment of the original in favour of comic action. Vanbrugh's two masterpieces still hold the stage and *The Confederacy* has been revived in recent years, but they are not produced as frequently as they deserve.

—Peter Lewis

---

**VILLIERS, George.   See BUCKINGHAM, 2nd Duke of.**

---

**WHITEHEAD, William.** English. Born in Cambridge, baptized 12 February 1715. Educated at Winchester College, 1729–35; Clare Hall, Cambridge (sizar), matriculated 1735, B.A. 1739, M.A. 1743. Fellow of Clare Hall from 1742; tutor to the future Earl of Jersey and Lord Villiers, 1745; gave up his fellowship, and settled in London, to devote himself to writing: quickly became known as poet and playwright; accompanied Villiers and Lord Nuneham on a tour of Germany and Italy, 1754–56; appointed Secretary and Registrar of the Order of Bath, 1756, and Poet Laureate, 1757; Reader of Plays for David Garrick, at Drury Lane, London, from 1762. *Died 14 April 1785.*

PUBLICATIONS

### Collections

*Plays and Poems.*   2 vols., 1774; revised edition, 3 vols., 1788.

### Plays

*The Roman Father,* from a play by Corneille (produced 1750).   1750.
*Fatal Constancy,* in *Poems on Several Occasions.*   1754.
*Creusa, Queen of Athens* (produced 1754).   1754.
*The School for Lovers,* from a play by Fontenelle (produced 1762).   1762.
*A Trip to Scotland* (produced 1770).   1770.

### Verse

*The Danger of Writing Verse.*   1741.
*Anne Boleyn to Henry the Eighth: An Epistle.*   1743.
*An Essay on Ridicule.*   1743.
*Atys and Adrastus: A Tale, in the Manner of Dryden's Fables.*   1744.
*On Nobility: An Epistle.*   1744.
*An Hymn to the Nymph of Bristol Spring.*   1751.
*Poems on Several Occasions.*   1754.
*Elegies, with an Ode to the Tiber.*   1757.
*Verses to the People of England.*   1758.
*A Charge to the Poets.*   1762.
*Variety: A Tale for Married People.*   1776.
*The Goat's Beard: A Fable.*   1777.

Reading List: *Whitehead, Poeta Laureatus* (in German) by August Bitter, 1933.

\*     \*     \*

William Whitehead began to write poetry during Pope's later years, but lived and wrote through the era variously known as the age of Pre-Romanticism, Reason, or Johnson. Most of the qualities implied by those associations can be found somewhere in his work. "The Enthusiast," for example, whose deism and nature description have been considered pre-romantic, is deeply indebted to the *Essay on Man*; the enthusiast for nature is finally taught that "man was made for man," and drawn from solitude to society. Many of his early poems pay their respects to Pope − verbally, ideologically, or both − and supply us with bad examples of late Augustan "definite-article verse" ("the vacant mind," "the social bosom," "the mutual morning task they ply"). Generally they are light, occasional, often epistolary, and gently satirical, when not congratulating the Royal Family on a marriage or birth. His commonest mood is mild, free-floating mockery, directed both at self and at a rather amusing environment. Whitehead publishes twelve quarto pages of heroic couplets under the title "The Danger of Writing Verse"; playfully emulates Spenser and the early Milton in the freely enjambed blank verse of *An Hymn to the Nymph of Bristol Spring*; and begins "The Sweepers" like a Johnson and Boswell joke: "I sing of Sweepers, frequent in thy streets,/ Augusta." Passion is seldom indulged and never intense, and Reason is often praised. The recurrent Tory patriotism was duly rewarded: as Laureate from 1757 to 1785, Whitehead had to compose birthday odes to George III throughout the American Revolution, a task he performed unflinchingly amid the customary howls of poets and critics.

Whitehead's interest in theatre began while he was a schoolboy at Winchester, where he played Marcia in a production of *Cato*, but reached new heights when the leading actor of the day took over Drury Lane in 1747. In "To Mr. Garrick" he warned the new manager – a nervous man anyway – that "A nation's taste depends on you/– Perhaps a nation's virtue too." The poem inaugurated a long association: Whitehead served as both playwright and play-reader for Drury Lane, and Garrick took leading roles in three of the poet's plays, all fairly successful. *The Roman Father*, a blank-verse tragedy based on Corneille's *Horace*, is distinctly reminiscent of *Cato*; the title-character Horatius (Garrick) is honoured to donate his sons' lives to Rome, and the closing paean to patriotism as the "first, best passion" was a sure clap-trap. Certain scenes, indeed, could be played as *parodies* of Addison, an idea which seems less far-fetched in view of *Fatal Constancy*, a fragmentary "sketch of a tragedy ... in the heroic taste." Though Whitehead gives only the hero's speeches and the scene directions, they are enough to suggest why he wrote no more tragedies after 1754. "My starting eyeballs hang/Upon her parting steps" cries the protagonist as his lover departs, after which they "Exeunt severally, languishing at each other." (Significantly, the play's forte is ingenious exits.) Unlike his plays designed for the stage, *Fatal Constancy* has the lightness of most of his verse, and a keen eye for theatrical absurdities. *Creusa, Queen of Athens*, with Garrick as Alestes, was produced to "great applause" and the approbation of Horace Walpole the same year.

Whitehead's only full-length comedy, *The School for Lovers*, caught and perpetuated the vogue of genteel or "sentimental" drama, though it also included stock bits of comic business that turn up in Goldsmith and Sheridan. The rhetoric of the prologue ("with strokes refin'd .../Formed on the classic scale his structures rise") conveys Whitehead's pure and reformist intentions as a playwright. *The Dramatic Censor* (1770) complained that "a dreadful soporific languor drowses over the whole, throwing both auditors and readers into a poppean lethargy," but the play, with Garrick as Dorilant, had a good first run and several revivals. Likewise *A Trip to Scotland*, Whitehead's only farce, pleased audiences for several seasons despite an unimpressive text. None of his plays reads well today, yet none failed, and *The Roman Father* and *The School for Lovers* were still being revived at the end of the eighteenth century.

—R. W. Bevis

---

**WILSON, John.**   English.   Born in London, baptized 27 December 1626; lived with his family in Plymouth, 1634–44. Educated at Exeter College, Oxford, matriculated 1644, but left without taking a degree; entered Lincoln's Inn, London, 1646; called to the Bar, 1652. Courtier and royalist: chairman of a board of sequestration after the Restoration; may have accompanied the Duke of Ormonde to Ireland, 1677; Recorder of Londonderry, 1681–89; possibly served as Secretary to the Viceroy of Ireland, 1687; lived in Dublin, 1689–90; returned to London, 1690. *Died c. 1695.*

PUBLICATIONS

Collections

*Dramatic Works,* edited by James Maidment and W. H. Logan.   1874.

Plays

> *The Cheats* (produced 1663). 1664; edited by Milton C. Nahm, 1935.
> *Andronicus Comnenius.* 1664.
> *The Protectors.* 1665.
> *Belphegor; or, The Marriage of the Devil* (produced 1675). 1691.

Verse

> *To His Grace James, Duke of Ormonde.* 1677.
> *To His Excellence Richard, Earl of Arran.* 1682.
> *A Pindaric to Their Sacred Majesties James II and Queen Mary on Their Joint Coronation.* 1685.

Other

> *A Discourse of Monarchy.* 1684.
> *Jus Regium Coronae.* 1688.

> Translator, *Moriae Encomium; or, The Praise of Folly,* by Erasmus. 1668.

Reading List: *Wilsons Dramen* by K. Faber, 1904; "John Wilson and 'Some Few Plays' " by Milton C. Nahm, in *Review of English Studies,* 1938.

\*      \*      \*

Like many of the more important Restoration dramatists, John Wilson devoted only a small part of his life to writing. In his case the crucial years were those immediately following the Restoration of the monarchy in 1660, when he wrote two prose comedies, *The Cheats* and *The Projectors*, a blank-verse tragedy, *Andronicus Comnenius*, and made his well-known translation of Erasmus's *Moriae Encomium* (*The Praise of Folly*). After the 1660's he wrote only one play, the tragi-comic *Belphegor* (performed in Dublin in 1675 and in London in 1690), and a few poems and tracts.

His reputation as a dramatist rests mainly on his first play, *The Cheats*, which was revived and reprinted from time to time during the rest of the seventeenth century and the first quarter of the eighteenth century. Wilson, a lawyer and a man of considerable learning, knew the work of Ben Jonson and his pre-Commonwealth followers intimately, and his two comedies belong to the Jonsonian comic tradition, especially to the "low" city comedy that Middleton specialized in; they therefore illustrate the element of continuity in seventeenth-century drama despite the closure of the theatres between 1642 and 1660. As comedies of "humours," both *The Cheats* and *The Projectors* contain numerous satirical portraits of the type found in the plays of Jonson and his "sons," as the names of the characters indicate; the cast of *The Projectors*, for example, includes Suckdry (a relative of Jonson's Volpone), Sir Gudgeon Credulous (very similar to Fitzdottrel in Jonson's *The Devil Is an Ass*), Jocose, Squeeze, and Leanchops. The world of Wilson's comedies is the familiar Jonsonian one of knaves and gulls, deceivers and deceived, cheats and cheated, and many of Wilson's targets, such as hypocrites, casuists, usurers, and misers, are identical to Jonson's. Derivative and backward-looking as Wilson's comedies are, they are lively and varied, and contain some memorable "humour" figures. Although *Belphegor* is a tragi-comedy set in Italy, it too shows Jonson's influence, being partly modelled on *The Devil Is an Ass*; Wilson's main source, however, is Machiavelli's version of a legend about a devil taking human form in order to discover the truth about women and marriage. In his one attempt at tragedy, *Andronicus Comnenius*, a study of a revengeful tyrant who indulges in wholesale slaughter to become Emperor of Constantinople, Wilson observes many of the neo-classical proprieties and rules, but is influenced by Shakespeare as well as Jonson, one scene being closely based on Richard's wooing of Anne in *Richard III*. Despite the abundance of off-stage action and murder, *Andronicus Comnenius* is a static play lacking in subtlety, and is much less interesting than Shakespeare's relatively immature history play about a similar character. Wilson's talent was for satirical comedy.

—Peter Lewis

---

**WYCHERLEY, William.**   English.   Born in Clive, near Shrewsbury, Shropshire, in 1640. Lived in Paris, 1655–60; spent a short time at Queen's College, Oxford (gentleman commoner), 1660; entered the Inner Temple, London, 1660, but never practised law. Married 1) the Countess of Drogheda in 1679 (died, 1681); 2) Elizabeth Jackson in 1715. Served in the Army, and may have been both an actor and theatre manager before he began to write for the theatre in 1671; enjoyed the patronage of Charles II until 1680 when the king banished him from court because of his marriage; gaoled for debt on his wife's estate, 1682: released and given a pension by James II, 1686; retired to Clive and devoted himself to writing poetry. *Died 31 December 1715.*

PUBLICATIONS

Collections

   *Complete Works*, edited by Montague Summers.   4 vols., 1924.
   *Complete Plays*, edited by Gerald Weales.   1967.

Plays

   *Love in a Wood; or, St. James's Park* (produced 1671).   1672.
   *The Gentleman Dancing-Master* (produced 1672).   1673.
   *The Country-Wife* (produced 1675).   1675; edited by David Cook and John Swannell, 1975.
   *The Plain-Dealer* (produced 1676).   1677.

Verse

   *Hero and Leander in Burlesque.*   1669.
   *Epistles to the King and Duke.*   1683.
   *Miscellany Poems.*   1704.
   *The Idleness of Business: A Satire.*   1705.
   *On His Grace the Duke of Marlborough.*   1707.

Other

*Posthumous Works,* edited by Lewis Theobald and Alexander Pope.   2 vols., 1729.


Reading List: *Wycherley: Sa Vie, Son Oeuvre* by Charles Perromat, 1921 (includes bibliography); *Brawny Wycherley* by Willard Connely, 1930; *Wycherley's Drama: A Link in the Development of English Satire* by Rose A. Zimbardo, 1965; *Wycherley* by P. F. Vernon, 1965; *Wycherley* by Katharine M. Rogers, 1972.


\*        \*        \*


Like so many literary gentlemen of the Restoration, William Wycherley fancied himself a poet, but it was not until he was in his sixties and the Restoration had begun to turn into the eighteenth century, spiritually as well as chronologically, that his *Miscellany Poems* appeared. The collection, in which long, tedious philosophic poems share space with love-and-seduction verses, is, as Macaulay said, "beneath criticism." Its publication did attract Alexander Pope, then a bright teen-ager on the literary make, who became a friend of the aging Wycherley. Pope's promise to polish the old man's verse was not kept during Wycherley's life, but it did lead to a volume, *Posthumous Works,* in which it is impossible to separate standard Wycherley from bad Pope. Wycherley occasionally dipped to prurience in his poems, as in "The Answer," a verse reply to "A Letter from Mr. Shadwell to Mr. Wycherley," but he seldom rose to the kind of wit that can be found on almost any page of *The Country-Wife.*

From the little we know about Wycherley, he was ambitious for social position and greedy for money but finally inept in his attempts to get what he wanted; he was also an urban snob as only a transplanted country boy can be. How so conventional a Restoration figure and so dull a poet could have written the comedies that mark him as one of the major English playwrights is still one of the mysteries of English literary history. We do not even know why he wrote them. He may have needed money; he may have wanted to impress the Restoration Wits – Rochester, Dorset, Sedley, Etherege – with whom he had become friends; he may have been overcome by a temporary artistic afflatus. For whatever reason, between 1671 and 1676, he wrote three good plays and one fine one, comedies that provide the theater's best and harshest view of Restoration society, and then, after the publication of *The Plain-Dealer* in 1677, he turned his back on the theater. He did return once, in 1696, to write a pedestrian prologue which was probably never performed for Catharine Trotter's preposterous *Agnes de Castro.* Strange company for the creator of Horner and Mrs. Pinchwife!

Wycherley's plays, like most of the Restoration comedies, are about the endless quest for sex and money, in and out of marriage, and the central theme is enriched by the playwright's marvelous sense for social pretension and polite hypocrisy. Whether he sends Alderman Gripe (*Love in a Wood*) into an old bawd's house, a pious prayer on his lips, or allows Lady Fidget (*The Country-Wife*) to reach from behind her prim exterior for the ever available Horner, he raises laughter at surface behavior which is the child of mendacious society by deep-seated lubricity. Except when a voice of pure delight, like that of the titular country wife, is needed to set off the shady machinations of most of the characters, there is no place for healthy sexuality in Wycherley's plays. Even Mrs. Pinchwife has to learn to deceive, but to her credit and to the play's advantage she remains a child trickster, the happy side of corruption. For the most part sex is a game (and often a brutal one) or a commodity (and often a shoddy one). From bawds and pimps to courting couples, Wycherley's characters know that sex is money, that whatever other entry marriage supplies, it opens purses. When Manly in *The Plain-Dealer* loses his jewels to the scheming Olivia, he is not simply robbed, he is unmanned.

Because Wycherley has always seemed so much a part of the world he depicts, some critics have taken Horner as an author surrogate and read the plays as a celebration of a society in which the true wits are successful manipulators, properly winning sex or money from the imperfect pretenders who deserve being used. Because that depicted world is essentially an ugly one, some critics have taken Manly as Wycherley (the playwright's later pseudonymous use of The Plain-Dealer in letters and in the preface to *Miscellany Poems* helped feed the notion) and taken Manly's abusive attacks on society as the playwright's true voice. There are obvious satiric elements in Wycherley's plays – conventional portraits of literary poseurs, bumbling cuckolds, overeager importers of foreign dress and manners – and they help prove the case for the concerned critic whether he sees Wycherley as Horner or Manly. On a deeper level, however, neither approach really works. On closer look, the clever Horner becomes a sex machine, servicing his clientele with all the efficiency and false gaiety of a fast-food shop, and Manly, who so hates hypocrisy, can be seen as a man for whom plain-dealing is a mask, a self-righteous, self-absorbed individual who uses the falseness of society as an excuse to act dishonestly. The strength of Wycherley's plays is that they are not ordinary period satires. He is the most modern of the Restoration writers because he refuses to provide a place for the audience to stand. His good characters, like Christina in *Love in a Wood*, turn fool through overstatement; his clever characters become butts; his fools refuse to remain skewered. John Dennis, praising Wycherley, once said " 'tis the Business of a Comick Poet to paint the Age in which he lives," and that Wycherley has done superbly, but without providing an ideational frame to fence in his presentation.

In emphasizing the ugliness of the world in which Wycherley's characters play their dead-serious games, I am in danger of falsifying the quality of the playwright's work, as have a number of recent revivals in which plain-dealing directors have displayed a chic fondness for sordid detail. Although the plays are harshly realistic in their approach to life, they are artificial in a theatrical sense. The characters are stereotypical and the exchanges between them are as set as vaudeville comic routines. Take, as an instance, the scene in *Love in a Wood* in which Dapperwit is about to introduce Ranger to his mistress, for whom he is pimping. The realistic content of the scene – the need to get the money in hand – need not interfere with the theatrical effect of a comic turn in which Dapperwit's loquacity, established in an earlier scene, becomes a hesitation device, enticing Ranger and then putting verbal obstacles in his path. Like so much that goes on in Wycherley's plays, this is overtly funny aside from any satirical implications; yet, unlike so much popular comedy, the theatrical fun of the scene does not disguise or weaken the essential nastiness of the situation. As though to emphasize the theatricality of his plays, Wycherley introduces in-jokes – references to his own work (*The Plain-Dealer*), to his actors (*The Gentleman Dancing-Master*), to the fact that the audience is in a theater. "She's come, as if she came expresly to sing the new Song she sung last night," says Hippolita in *The Gentleman Dancing-Master*, and a character who has no other function in the play walks on stage to perform a number. This kind of playfulness not only underscores the conscious artifice in Wycherley's work, it reminds the audience that there is a distance between the action and its referent, that these very funny plays are about a world in which the comic stereotypes have painful counterparts. Only occasionally, as when the brutality of Manly threatens the comic surface of *The Plain-Dealer*, does the real world come dragging its unpleasantness onto the stage. For the most part, Wycherley invokes laughter haunted by a suspicion which, a beat or two beyond the laugh, asks what was so funny. At his best, which means at almost any point in *The Country-Wife*, the laughter and the questioning come at the same time, the play's artistry and its documentary integrity go hand-in-hand.

—Gerald Weales

---

# NOTES ON CONTRIBUTORS

**ASHLEY, Leonard R. N.** Professor of English, Brooklyn College, City University of New York. Author of *Colley Cibber*, 1965; *19th-Century British Drama*, 1967; *Authorship and Evidence · A Study of Attribution and the Renaissance Drama*, 1968; *History of the Short Story*, 1968; *George Peele · The Man and His Work*, 1970. Editor of the *Enriched Classics* series, several anthologies of fiction and drama, and a number of facsimile editions. **Essays:** Henry Brooke; Colley Cibber; Aaron Hill; Edward Moore; Elkanah Settle.

**BACKSCHEIDER, Paula R.** Associate Professor of English, University of Rochester, New York. Author of "Defoe's Women: Snares and Prey" in *Studies in Eighteenth Century Culture*, 1977, and "Home's *Douglas* and the Theme of the Unfulfilled Life" in *Studies in Scottish Literature*, 1978. Editor of the Garland series *Eighteenth-Century Drama* (60 vols.) and of *Probability, Time, and Space in Eighteenth Century Literature*, 1978. **Essay:** John Crowne.

**BATTESTIN, Martin C.** William R. Kenan, Jr., Professor of English, University of Virginia, Charlottesville. Author of *The Moral Basis of Fielding's Art*, 1959, *The Providence of Wit · Aspects of Form in Augustan Literature and the Arts*, 1974, and a forthcoming biography of Fielding. Editor of the Wesleyan Edition of Fielding's works, and of *Joseph Andrews*, *Tom Jones*, and *Amelia*. **Essay:** Henry Fielding.

**BEVIS, R. W.** Member of the Department of English, University of British Columbia, Vancouver. Editor, *Eighteenth Century Drama · Afterpieces*, 1970. **Essays:** George Colman, the Elder; John Dennis; Samuel Foote; Charles Macklin; William Whitehead.

**FAULKNER, Peter.** Member of the Department of English, University of Exeter, Devon. Author of *William Morris and W. B. Yeats*, 1962; *Yeats and the Irish Eighteenth Century*, 1965; *Humanism in the English Novel*, 1976; *Modernism*, 1977. Editor of *William Morris · The Critical Heritage*, 1973, and of works by Morris. **Essay:** Thomas Holcroft.

**HILSON, J. C.** Lecturer in English, University of Leicester. Editor of *Augustan Worlds* (with M. M. B. Jones and J. R. Watson), 1978, and *An Essay on Historical Composition*, by James Moor, 1978. Author of articles on Hume, Richardson, Smollett, and Conrad. **Essay:** Roger Boyle, Earl of Orrery.

**HUGHES, Leo.** Professor of English, University of Texas, Austin. Author of *A Century of English Farce*, 1956, and *The Drama's Patrons*, 1971. Editor of *Ten English Farces* (with Arthur H. Scouten), 1948, and *The Plain Dealer* by William Wycherley, 1967. **Essay:** Edward Ravenscroft.

**JEFFARES, A. Norman.** Professor of English Studies, University of Stirling, Scotland; Editor of *Ariel · A Review of International English Literature*, and General Editor of the Writers and Critics series and the New Oxford English series; Past Editor of *A Review of English Studies*. Author of *Yeats · Man and Poet*, 1949; *Seven Centuries of Poetry*, 1956; *A Commentary on the Collected Poems* (1958) and *Collected Plays* (1975) *of Yeats*. Editor of *Restoration Comedy*, 1974, and *Yeats · The Critical Heritage*, 1977. **Essays:** William Congreve; Richard Brinsley Sheridan.

**KELLY, Gary.** Member of the Department of Engiish, University of Alberta, Edmonton. Author of *The English Jacobin Novel 1780–1805*, 1976. Editor of *Mary, and The Wrongs of Women* by Mary Wollstonecraft, 1976. **Essay:** Elizabeth Inchbald.

**KUNZ, Don.** Associate Professor of English, University of Rhode Island, Kingston. Author of *The Drama of Thomas Shadwell*, 1972, and of articles on Shadwell in *Restoration and Eighteenth Century Theatre Research.* **Essay:** Thomas Shadwell.

**LEWIS, Peter.** Lecturer in English, University of Durham. Author of *The Beggar's Opera* (critical study), 1976, and articles on Restoration and Augustan drama and modern poetry. Editor of *The Beggar's Opera* by John Gay, 1973, and *Poems '74* (anthology of Anglo-Welsh poetry), 1974. **Essays:** George Farquhar; John Gay; George Lillo; Sir John Vanbrugh; John Wilson.

**LINK, Frederick M.** Professor of English, University of Nebraska, Lincoln. Author of *Aphra Behn*, 1968, and *English Drama 1660–1800 · A Guide to Information Sources*, 1976. Editor of *The Rover* by Behn, 1967, and *Aureng-Zebe* by John Dryden, 1971. **Essays:** Aphra Behn; Henry Carey; Hannah Cowley.

**MACKERNESS, E. D.** Member of the Department of English Literature, University of Sheffield. Author of *The Heeded Voice · Studies in the Literary Status of the Anglican Sermon 1830–1900*, 1959, *A Social History of English Music*, 1964, and *Somewhere Further North · A History of Music in Sheffield*, 1974. Editor of *The Journals of George Sturt 1890–1927*, 1967. **Essay:** John Hughes.

**MALEK, James S.** Professor of English and Associate Graduate Dean, University of Idaho, Moscow. Author of *The Arts Compared · An Aspect of Eighteenth-Century British Aesthetics*, 1974, and of articles in *Modern Philology, The Journal of Aesthetics and Art Criticism, Neuphilologische Mitteilungen, Texas Studies in Literature and Language,* and other periodicals. **Essays:** Sir George Etherege; John Home; Arthur Murphy.

**MINER, Earl.** Townsend Martin Professor of English and Comparative Literature, Princeton University, New Jersey. Author of *Dryden's Poetry*, 1967; *An Introduction to Japanese Court Poetry*, 1968; *The Metaphysical Mode from Donne to Cowley*, 1969; *The Cavalier Mode from Jonson to Cotton*, 1971; *Seventeenth-Century Imagery*, 1971; *The Restoration Mode from Milton to Dryden*, 1974; *Japanese Linked Poetry*, 1978. **Essay:** John Dryden.

**MORPURGO, J. E.** Professor of American Literature, University of Leeds. Author and editor of many books, including the *Pelican History of the United States*, 1955 (third edition, 1970), and volumes on Cooper, Lamb, Trelawny, Barnes Wallis, and on Venice, Athens, and rugby football. **Essay:** John Burgoyne.

**OLIVER-MORDEN, B. C.** Teacher at the Open University and the University of Keele. Editor of the 18th-Century section of *The Year's Work in English 1973.* **Essay:** Oliver Goldsmith.

**ROGERS, Pat.** Professor of English, University of Bristol. Author of *Grub Street · Studies in a Subculture*, 1972, and *The Augustan Vision*, 1974. Editor of *A Tour Through Great Britain* by Daniel Defoe, 1971, *Defoe · The Critical Heritage*, 1972, and *The Eighteenth Century*, 1978. **Essay:** Susanna Centlivre.

**SCOUTEN, Arthur H.** Professor of English, University of Pennsylvania, Philadelphia. Author of articles on Swift, Defoe, and the London theatre in periodicals. Editor of *Ten English Farces* (with Leo Hughes), 1948, *The London Stage 3*, 2 vols., 1961, and *1*, 1965, and *A Bibliography of the Writings of Swift* by Teerink Herman, second edition, 1963. **Essays:** John Banks; Thomas D'Urfey; Sir Robert Howard; Nathaniel Lee.

**SOLOMON, Harry M.** Associate Professor of English, Auburn University, Alabama. Author of *Sir Richard Blackmore* (forthcoming), and of articles on Shaftesbury, Swift, and others for *Southern Humanities Review, Keats-Shelley Journal, Studies in English Literature,* and other periodicals. **Essay:** Robert Dodsley.

**SPENCER, Christopher.** Professor of English, University of North Carolina, Greensboro. Author of *Nahum Tate,* 1972. Editor of *Davenant's Macbeth from the Yale Manuscript,* 1961, and *Five Restoration Adaptations of Shakespeare,* 1965. **Essay:** Nahum Tate.

**STAGG, Louis Charles.** Professor of English, Memphis State University, Tennessee; Member of the Executive Committee, Tennessee Philological Association. Author of *Index to Poe's Critical Vocabulary,* 1966; *Index to the Figurative Language in the Tragedies of Webster, Jonson, Heywood, Chapman, Marston, Tourneur,* and *Middleton,* 7 vols., 1967–70, revised edition, as *Index to the Figurative Language of the Tragedies of Shakespeare's Chief 17th-Century Contemporaries,* 1977. **Essay:** Nicholas Rowe.

**STROUP, Thomas B.** Professor Emeritus, University of Kentucky, Lexington. Author of a book on composition, and of *Microcosmos · The Shape of the Elizabethan Play,* 1965, and *Religious Rite and Ceremony in Milton's Poetry,* 1968. Editor or Joint Editor of *Humanistic Scholarship in the South,* 1948; *South Atlantic Studies for Sturgis E. Leavitt,* 1953; *The Works of Nathaniel Lee,* 2 vols., 1954–55; *The Selected Poems of George Daniel of Beswick,* 1959; *The Cestus · A Mask,* 1962; *The University and the American Future,* 1965; *The Humanities and the Understanding of Reality,* 1966. **Essay:** Thomas Otway.

**TASCH, Peter A.** Associate Professor of English, Temple University, Philadelphia; Co-Editor of *The Scriblerian.* Author of *The Dramatic Cobbler · The Life and Works of Isaac Bickerstaff,* 1971. Editor of *Fables by the Late Mr. Gay,* 1970. **Essays:** Isaac Bickerstaff; Charles Dibdin; David Garrick; Hugh Kelly.

**THOMSON, Peter.** Professor of Drama, University of Exeter, Devon. Author of *Ideas in Action,* 1977. Editor of *Julius Caesar* by Shakespeare, 1970; *Essays on Nineteenth-Century British Theatre* (with Kenneth Richards), 1971; *The Eighteenth-Century English Stage,* 1973; *Lord Byron's Family,* 1975. **Essays:** George Colman, the Younger; Thomas Morton; John O'Keeffe.

**THORNTON, Ralph R.** Associate Professor of English, La Salle College, Philadelphia. Editor of *The Wives' Excuse,* 1973, and *The Maid's Last Prayer,* 1978, both by Thomas Southerne. **Essay:** Thomas Southerne.

**TRUSSLER, Simon.** Editor of *Theatre Quarterly.* Theatre Critic, *Tribune,* 1969–76. Author of several books on theatre and drama, including studies of John Osborne, Arnold Wesker, John Whiting, Harold Pinter, and Edward Bond, and of articles on theatre bibliography and classification. Editor of two collections of eighteenth-century plays and of *The Oxford Companion to the Theatre,* 1969. **Essays:** Richard Cumberland; Sir Richard Steele; George Villiers, Duke of Buckingham.

**WEALES, Gerald.** Professor of English, University of Pennsylvania, Philadelphia; Drama Critic for *The Reporter* and *Commonweal.* Author of *Religion in Modern English Drama,* 1961; *American Drama since World War II,* 1962; *A Play and Its Parts,* 1964; *The Jumping-Off Place · American Drama in the 1960's,* 1969; *Clifford Odets,* 1971. Editor of *The Complete Plays of William Wycherley,* 1966, and, with Robert J. Nelson, of the collections *Enclosure,* 1975, and *Revolution,* 1975. **Essay:** William Wycherley.